I0447369

How to Permanently Reset Your Body Weight Set Point

Ray Blais

How to Permanently Reset Your Body Weight Set Point

Copyright © 2016-2017 by Ray Blais and The Transformation Center

All rights reserved. No part of this book may be reproduced or transmitted in any form or by any means without written permission from the author.

ISBN-13: 978-1541216174

ISBN-10: 1541216172

Table of Contents

Is This Book For You?

I don't wish to waste anybody's time or hard-earned money. This is not a "fluff piece," and I will not be "tickling" your ears by telling you what I think you want to hear. Losing weight **PERMANENTLY** is not complicated, and in fact, it's a lot simpler than most people realize. Unfortunately, people unknowingly start to **<u>FIGHT against themselves</u>**. Your body is incredibly well-designed and very capable of dropping all the extra fat. You just need to get out of its way and stop fighting against it. Research has repeatedly shown how to effectively lose weight. The biggest problem is that the health, fitness, and supplement industry lose most of their profits when you do it properly. Can you imagine what would happen to these industries if everyone kept their New Year's resolutions? Do you think they all have your best interests in mind?

If you:
- Hate shopping for clothes,
- Are ashamed when having sex,
- Don't believe your spouse's compliments,
- Are tired of not being able to "keep up,"
- Know you're not setting a good example for your kids
- Sincerely want to make a change...

Then this book is indeed for you.

However, if you're looking for a quick fix, a Band-Aid solution, a few secret tricks that will "back-fire" in a few weeks, then this book is NOT for you.

I'm hoping you are serious, that you want to raise your life to a new level and that you want successful and permanent weight loss. Anything less, and you might as well save your money.

Want a bit more information? Flip over a few pages to "What's this book about."

Dedication

To my wife, Lise, for supporting me through all my crazy ideas and running our home in a way that has allowed me to chase my dreams.

Also, to all my students and everybody else that has tried so many times and so many ways of losing stubborn FAT. While working with thousands of students over the last 13 years, I have listened to so many "stories" of the constant pain and struggle overweight people endure every day. This is unimaginable to someone that has not experienced this issue personally. Unfortunately, there is so much misinformation and conflict of interest out there, that it's difficult to sort the fluff from the cold hard facts. The war is NOT lost! With new weapons and information at your disposal, perhaps one last battle is all that's needed.

To your permanent and sustainable success,

Ray

Disclaimer

This program is for educational and informative purposes only and is not intended as medical or professional advice. Always consult your doctor before making any changes to your diet or nutrition program. The use of diet and nutrition to control metabolic disorders and disease is a very complicated science, and is not the purpose of this program.

No health claims are made for this program. This nutrition and exercise program will not help cure, heal, or correct any illness, metabolic disorder, or medical condition. The author is not a medical doctor, registered dietitian, or clinical nutritionist; the author is a fitness and nutrition consultant and coach.

If you have diabetes, chronic hypertension, high blood cholesterol, cardiovascular disease, or any other medical condition or metabolic disorder requiring special nutritional considerations, we suggest you consult a healthcare professional.

Your nutrition plan will not be effective by itself. You must combine a good diet with an appropriate exercise program for optimal results. If you have been sedentary and are unaccustomed to vigorous exercise, you should obtain your physician's clearance before beginning an exercise program.

The author and publisher shall have neither liability nor responsibility to any person or entity with respect to any of the information contained in this book. The user assumes all risk for any injury, loss, or damage caused or alleged to be caused, directly or indirectly by using any information described in this course.

The following information is an oversimplification as the processes that maintain hunger, digestion, and metabolism are incredibly complex and not entirely understood. There are a myriad of different checks and balances that CONTINUALLY affect our set points.

It All Starts Here

Life is won or lost
in your mind FIRST.

Ray Blais

Careful, you can expect hard-hitting, "raw" information whenever you see the following:

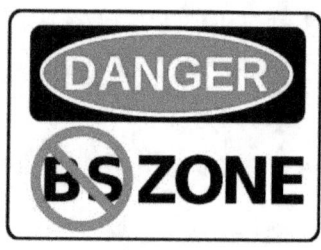

In a world of "political correctness at all cost" and "don't risk offense..." what follows this sign can catch people off guard.

Those who are constantly looking to make something offensive or seeking scapegoats to absolve themselves of personal responsibility will **NOT** enjoy these "danger" sections.

Those serious about improving their lives will read and pay close attention.

Always remember: those who play victim, give away their power.

Instead, grab life "by the horns" and start designing the life you deserve!

"You are 100% responsible."

About the Transformation Center

The Transformation Center is part of the Family Kickboxing club. Founded in 2004, the club filled the need for kickboxing in Sudbury and the surrounding areas. UFC was mostly unheard of still, and I had to travel to North Bay three times a week for training. (260 km round trip). This was very time consuming, especially during the northern Ontario winter months. On hearing that my coach was moving to Sudbury, I jumped at the chance and opened the club.

Through the years, the club's focus has changed very little. That focus is to bring out the best out in every student.

Despite the name of our club, the emphasis has never been just on excelling at kickboxing. It has always been so much more.

The two areas that we concentrate and focus on are:

#1 - Health, fitness, weight management, etc.

#2 - Personal growth, expansion of comfort zones, increased self-confidence, improved self-image, etc.

I concentrate on things like self-confidence and self-image because throughout the years, I have watched far too many people focus simply on "losing weigh" at the expense of their "inner-man." The end result is usually short-term at best, and nearly nothing at worst. You may physically lose that extra 50 pounds, but in the end, if your subconscious mind and your self-image still perceives you as being that over-weight person, it's ALL coming back along with a few extra pounds for good measure!

Just losing weight is NOT that complicated.

Losing it PERMANENTLY is a whole different story.

With this book, my goal is to help you with that.

The Transformation Center – Family Kickboxing
www.familykickboxing.net

What This Book
Is About...

Hi, my name is Ray Blais.

I wanted to introduce myself a bit before we get started so I could let you know what this book is about, and more importantly, what it's not about, and what you will get out of it.

First, this book is not about what might work if you had unwavering self-discipline, a lot of time, special and expensive equipment, or had access to "new" wonder supplements, etc. Not remotely.

This book is not filled with endless "case studies" to help fill the pages, ongoing babble with fictional stories, or countless "opinions" and unsubstantiated mumbo-jumbo.

My goal is to give you the cold, hard facts, the tools and proven strategies that you can put to work immediately and start reaping the results you want. Permanent results.

Unfortunately, in order to do that, I will have to shoot down a few of the favorite "sacred cows," beliefs that in the short term may appear to be accurate and productive but have PROVEN without a doubt to fail 99.9% of the time in the long run.

By stripping away all the nonsense, we are left with what has always worked. Our bodies and minds are incredibly well-designed and are more than capable of taking care of themselves IF we get out of the way.

This book will take you step-by-step, in the right order, at the correct pace, and send you on your way to permanent weight loss. From the first section, we will start creating a firm foundation with Decisions, Clarity, and Belief, and then move forward to destroying nine of the most destructive and harmful weight loss myths that trip so many well-intentioned people up. We'll tackle why our cravings are so powerful, and how to effectively deal with them in both the short term and the long term. Next, we'll learn how to properly and permanently "reset" your body weight. Finally, we'll deal with the one piece of the puzzle that's always missing: your mind. When you lose weight physically and it's not accompanied with a matching self-image or similar mental shift, it will ALWAYS come back, and usually with a few "friends.

If you are serious, I agree to being your long-distance coach. It doesn't matter if you're half way around the world or if you're here working out in my facilities. I would be giving you the same information and following the same steps.

What works, works.

To your success,

Ray Blais
Head coach

Chapter One:
Breaking Free From Your Weight Loss Prison

The Three Dynamos

"Decision, Clarity, and Belief," the Three Dynamos, are some of the most powerful success principles available to us. There's no magic tricks involved, and there's nothing complicated about them. They've been proven time and again over thousands of years. All successful people, in all walks of life, have and continue to use these whether they realize it or not.

THEY WORK EVERYTIME

Before we begin...

If you've somehow found yourself in the "Weight Loss Prison" or worse yet, you've been there for several years, then we have some serious work ahead of us.

The first thing you need to do BEFORE everything else, is to take some time and be alone with your thoughts. A quiet walk maybe? Myself, I like to do my thinking while riding on a quiet road, my favorite being Hwy 637 to Kilarney.

Take some time and contemplate your past, your present, and your future as it relates to your health and weight. In today's world, many go at great lengths to AVOID having to think at all! Was your first thought, "I don't have time?"

Seriously, are you "defeated" before you even get started? Will you rush into this like you did all the other failed attempts? Ending your efforts with thoughts like, "I knew **IT** wouldn't work…"

Well, "this" isn't going to work either if you don't do it properly.

Since you're taking the time to actually read this book, then you're already way ahead of the pack. I will assume you are serious, and I hope my assumptions about you are correct.

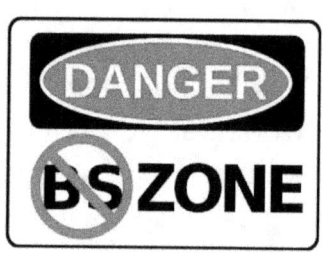

Let me be really blunt here. Unless you take the time here and do some soul searching, NOTHING will ever work. If you're finding yourself in this Weight Loss Prison, then NOTHING you've done in the past has worked! It doesn't matter if you did that "cleanse" or that "no carb" diet or whatever and lost X amount of pounds. If you put it all back on, news flash, it didn't work!

IT DIDN'T WORK!

Will this be a "repeat?" Same old, same old? I really hope not. I have extended my hand here, and I am willing to help and work with all who are serious about putting their lives back on track.

But it all begins with you. Agree with me that this is a BIG deal. Being overweight affects every area of your life (including your children).

It all begins with you realizing that this is a big undertaking.

So please, start by taking some quality time for yourself. Some quiet time to look at the big picture. Resist all judgements. Just look at where you've been on this FAT issue. How long has it been? How does the whole thing make you feel? Take a few minutes and think back at all the different "ways and things" you've done in the past to try and permanently lose weight. If you want to significantly increase your odds of success this time, why not do it properly? It all starts here:

#1 - List the TOP EIGHT ways that being fat hurts you.

#2 - List the TOP TWO ways being fat hurts those around you.

#3 - List the SINGLE, most emotionally charged benefit you will get from winning this weight loss battle once and for all. (Just ONE, the biggie.)

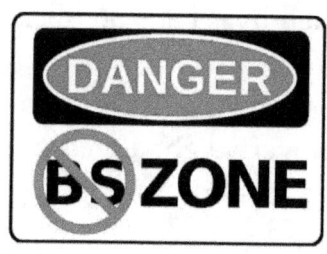

If my saying, "...eight ways that being fat hurts you," happens to offends you, then it is important that you ask yourself WHY it offends you!

When I ask these three questions to my Weight Loss Challenge (WLC) participants, I get a variety of reactions. Many take this short assignment, and they think it will be a "breeze." However, when they really start thinking of all the ways being overweight hurts them and those around them, they are shocked. On many occasions, WLC participants tell me that they've tried several times to do the exercise and tears start running down their faces as it dawns on them how serious this all is.

Here are a few examples of what I've been told...

"...it hurts my relationship with my husband in that I don't believe him when he says I'm pretty..."

"...hurts my friends because I cannot keep up and do certain activities with them..."

"...hurts my relationship because I am ashamed of my body when we have sex..."

"...I absolutely hate trying on clothes..."

"...it hurts my daughter because she wants to play, and I'm having to find excuses because I just can't..."

When you stop and really think about how serious this all is, a foundation is being set for your weight loss success. Without this solid foundation, even the best of your intentions and efforts will fail.

So I must insist that you take or MAKE the time and answer the three questions. The more specific and detailed you are, the more honest with yourself even if it hurts, the better your chances of success. Go ahead. Nobody will read your answers. It's between you and you alone. Grab a pen and a note pad.

Make yourself a cup of coffee or something, and do yourself a favor: do the exercise. Don't cheat yourself of the life you are capable of living. Stop and do this. You owe it to yourself.

Assuming you've followed through, that you did the exercise properly and honestly, then a big huge **congratulations** to you. You are in the top 3% of the population, and you are a perfect candidate for success. If you haven't, if you're already taking short cuts... what can I say? You most likely took short cuts in the past, and how has that worked out for you?

> "Without a clear **vision**, you don't have a **destination**. Without a **destination**, you have no **direction**. Without **direction**, you're stuck where you are!"

So let's make sure we KNOW where we've been and where we are heading.

The Power of Decision

Let the fun begin. Although many might be tempted to skip directly to **Chapter Four, "Resetting Your Body Weight Set Point,"** that would be a mistake. The reason is simple: absolutely NOTHING GETS DONE without first making a quality decision. I mean, you won't even read this book unless you make a decision to do so. Have a quick look back in your life. EVERYTHING, both good and bad, came from making decisions. And yes, even avoiding to make a decision IS A DECISION! To me, it's pretty simple. True POWER begins with "deciding." No matter what area of your life we are talking about, making decisions is where the real power begins.

> "It is our decisions and not our condition that determine the quality of our lives."
> Tony Robbins

What **you** decide TODAY will determine where you end up tomorrow. What **you** decide today regarding your body will determine how you look tomorrow. Tomorrow will surely arrive, and it will be a direct result of all your decisions. Today is when **you** decide what your tomorrow will be, what it will look like. It is all in your hands. It is all in your power; your power of **CHOICE**. It doesn't matter how many things you've tried or how many times you've tried them. Today is a new day, and with this book in your hands, along with a bit of time and some effort, you have all the knowledge and tools necessary for success except for one small item. You still must make a decision. You have to decide, are you going to **learn** and **do** what has to be learnt and done in order to reach your goal, in order to lose the fat once and for all? Permanently?

> Different decisions precede different actions. Different actions precede different results.

We will be making some important decisions in a few minutes. These decisions will have an enormous impact on whether you succeed or fail. These decisions will determine how and what you look like in the coming months and years, what you're able or not able to do, how much "LIFE" you will be able to enjoy. These decisions will affect your health, your confidence, your self-image, how others look at you, what others think about you, and much more importantly, how you think of yourself.

So what truly precedes how you will look and feel tomorrow? What you will be deciding today.

While I'm at it, here are two short passages from one of the greatest books ever written (in my opinion), *Awaken The Giant Within* by Tony Robbins.

> "You see, it's not what's happening to you now or what has happened in your past that determines who you become. Rather, it's in your decisions about what to focus on, what things mean to you, and what you're going to

do about them that will determine your ultimate destiny." (Robbins, pg. 40)

Here's another one from the same book:

The Niagara Syndrome

"In fact, most people live what I call 'The Niagara Syndrome.' I believe that life is like a river, and that most people jump on the river of life without ever really deciding where they want to end up. So, in a short period of time, they get caught up in the current: current events, current fears and current challenges. When they come to forks in the river, they don't consciously decide where they want to go, or which is the right direction for them. They merely 'go with the flow.' They become a part of the mass of people who are directed by the environment instead of by their own values. As a result, they feel out of control. They remain in this unconscious state until one day the sound of raging water awakens them, and they discover that they're five feet from Niagara Falls in a boat with no oars. At this point, they say, 'Oh, shoot!' But by then it's too late. They're going to take a fall. Sometimes it's an emotional fall. Sometimes it's a physical fall. Sometimes it's a financial fall. **It's likely that whatever challenges you have in your life**

> **currently could have been avoided by some better decisions upstream."** (Robbins, pg. 41)

Powerful words indeed! I read that passage several times every year. It's so easy to fall prey to the "Niagara Syndrome," so we must always be on the lookout for this. Whenever "things" are not going the way we'd planned, a quick look back will help us realize where we "slacked-off" with our purposeful decision making.

The fact is we can accomplish just about anything in life if we:

> #1 - Clearly decide what we want
> #2 - Take massive action
> #3 - Notice what's working and what's not
> #4 - Adjust whatever needs adjusting

So what exactly is this big decision that is so important?

It's your honest, well thought out decision that you will do whatever it takes to lose this weight <u>properly, correctly,</u> once and for all. You will not try to take the easy way out, the so called short-cuts. That you will resist thinking that it "won't work," that "you can't do it," that "it's in your genes," or a hundred other self-defeating thoughts that simply aren't true.

This has been done successfully by thousands of everyday regular folks just like you, many who train at our facility.

This is your time. Will you make the decision right now?

Decide today.

> "There are a thousand excuses for failure but never a good reason."
>
> Mark Twain

The Power of Clarity

One of the most important words in your success vocabulary is "Clarity." This word should be way, way ahead of "hard work, discipline, sacrifice," etc. It should be found right after "decision."

> "Do it or don't do it, but don't make excuses."
>
> Brian Tracy

Once you've properly made a decision, you must then start clarifying it. Look around, talk to successful people, talk to everyday people about the area they are successful in. You will notice a common theme.

You will also notice the same theme in areas of failure. Successful individuals are very CLEAR about what they want, where they're going, why they want it, the work or effort they're willing to trade for it, etc. They can describe exactly "HOW, WHAT, WHY, and WHERE." They have clarity.

Even everyday people, people you wouldn't classify as successful, can have a hobby that they're very successful at. Take gardening as an example. These people may be failing miserably in all other areas of their lives, but talk to them about gardening. You will soon see why they are successful. They have already planned what they will plant next year, how much they'll plant, where in the garden, they know how, what, and where. They have COMPLETE CLARITY about their next year's gardening plans.

What does failure have in common with success? Since most of us don't view ourselves as a failure, let me rephrase this as: "the areas in our lives that are not where we'd like them to be." What is the common theme? <u>May I suggest a complete lack of clarity?</u> There is no planning, no goals, no clear picture, no date or time line, no calculated cost, etc.

Now let's tie this in with weight loss. Ask just about anybody that cares about themselves and has a weight issue, and they'll quickly admit that they should probably lose a few pounds. Better yet, they'd really like to lose a few pounds. Most of them have NOT taken the first step, which is to make a DECISION. Even assuming they've made a decision to lose weight... that's about just as far as 90% of the people get. That goes a long way towards "why" only a small percentage lose weight permanently.

Ask the average weight loss challenge participant what they want and how they're going to get it, and you'll probably get something like, "I want to lose as much as I can by doing these workouts for the next two months." Unfortunately, that won't get you very far. If that's all there was to it, then everyone would look awesome.

Let me ask you a few questions:

- How much are you going to lose?
- In what time frame?
- How will you achieve this?
- What exercise program will you use?
- What changes will you implement with your diet?
- What is your game plan for overcoming:
  o Cravings?
  o Temptations?
  o Low blood sugar?
  o Slowing metabolism?
  o Social gatherings?
  o Your emotional triggers?
  o Muscle wasting (loss)?

- o Low energy?
- o Disappearing motivation?
- o Decreasing strength?
- o Constipation?
- o Scheduling issues?
- o Negative self-talk?
- o Mood swings?
- o Etc.!

Now you're getting a glimpse as to why upwards of 90% of people fail when it comes to weight loss. They have no CLARITY. They are "winging it." Unfortunately, that has never worked in the past, and it's NOT about to. You can "really" want it; you can "really" work hard at it. But that alone won't work either. You've tried that before, probably several times. How did it work out for you? What makes you think "this" time will be different?

Let's Be Clear

Successful weight loss belongs to those that grab the whole process with both hands and with both eyes wide open. It belongs to those that will take actions other than just "hope and pray," rather than just "try." This drastic change means investing in yourself and in your education. No one else will do it for you, and you can't act on information you've yet to learn. So let's get very clear about what we want to accomplish in the coming weeks. Let's look at the big question: "Why?"

You've already taken the first step. You've made the first move. You're already miles ahead of the masses. You actually made a DECISION to lose weight. Now we need to know **WHY?**

The road ahead is full of twists and turns, and it's going to get bumpy along the way. Once you start pushing against the lower boundaries of your natural body weight set point, we will start facing some battles in which the going could get rough. If you don't have a good enough "why" to back up your decision, you'll be in big trouble.

> "A big enough WHY will always overcome and find the HOWs."

Here we go

You need to know WHY you want to lose weight. Properly done, this will be extremely personal. You need to dig down deep and get the real emotional reasons. It is "emotion" that runs the majority of our lives. Again: why do you want to lose weight? How will it make you feel? How do you feel now?

27

Examples of "whys" that are completely **devoid of any power.**

I want to lose weight because...

- I will feel better.
- I will look better.
- I will be able to play with my kids.
- I will fit in my dress.
- I won't be so tired.
- I should.
- My spouse wants me to.
- For my health.
- Etc.

These are all useless. **They have no emotional drive or fire.** They don't "light" or stir you up. They definitely won't help you power through the rough spots, the hard times.

The first disagreement that pops up with your spouse, you will say, "The heck with it!"

The next time you're tired you'll just say, "I have to eat..."

The next time you're down in the dumps... out comes the ice cream or chocolate.

The next time you're tired after playing with the kids, you'll just say, "Well, I'm not a kid anymore."

You need some real fire in your answer. You need it to be loaded with <u>emotional energy</u>. Again, this is all very personal. Only you will see your answers. Only you will know all this. Only you can dig this deep within yourself.

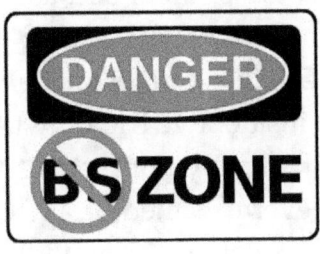

Remember, having it in our head is NOT GOOD ENOUGH. If you can't do this simple exercise, there's absolutely no way you'll be able to handle the challenges that come with losing weight successfully. You are wasting everybody's time. Oops, did that hurt? If yes, I'm so sorry... blah blah blah, grow some skin! (See, that's EMOTION, and I may have stirred some in you.) You are about to enter a serious battle. You will need to toughen up mentally and emotionally. You are doing this for YOU, and this time YOU will be successful. You will come out of this tougher, stronger, and ready to conquer even more "territory" in other areas of your life. Many have already done it, and now it's your time.

> "Losers make excuses;
> winners make progress."
> Brian Tracy

So here is an example of a good WHY answer. **This is clarity.**

> I need to lose 35 pounds because I'm 32 and still single. There's this hot guy at work. I mean, whenever he walks by I just get all nervous, and I kinda shake inside. I've tried my best to get his attention, but he barely notices me. This guy is everything I've ever dreamed of. I need to "pull it together" and lose about 35 pounds. I know he will notice me then. At that weight I would have a good shot. I'm tired of being single. My friends are all… and I'm starting to get lonely…

Now this person means business. You can feel the emotions so much that some people might feel compelled to jump in and "defend" being single. Keep in mind this is just one person's answer. It's not a matter of right or wrong. It's a matter of the honest truth as it relates to you. For this person, overcoming problems along the way will be a breeze, which is especially true if she uses a few smart strategies, like putting his picture on the fridge.

Some want to lose weight because they've experienced one too many embarrassing moments. Their health is failing. They can't keep up with their friends, and this has slowly changed them. They now have two asthma pumps, and the doctor says they're borderline diabetic. Do you hate shopping for clothes? Do you believe your spouse when they tell you that you are pretty? Dig deep down. Honestly, how do you feel when you are naked, the lights are on, and you're not alone?

There are all kinds of reasons, and yours is the truth for you. The only wrong reasons are the "weak" reasons, because THEY ARE NOT TRUE.

One last comment on this. When looking for your own personal "why do I want to lose weight..." truth, **you have to dig DEEP**. It goes something like this:

Why do you want to lose weight?

Because I want to look better.

Why do you want to look better?

Because I don't like the way I look.

Why don't you like the way you look?

Are you kidding? Look at me.

Why don't you like the way you look?

Because I feel unattractive.

Why do you feel unattractive?

Because I can't fit in my nice clothes, and when I move around I feel like a _____.

Then you start over.

What else don't you like about your current condition? Why?

This all takes time and effort. It's not an easy exercise because it forces you to face certain things about your life that are usually kept buried deep, and for obvious reasons, people are naturally afraid to deal with these things. We are so used to telling ourselves lies.

Just last night, I was talking with a student. The conversation was very pleasant. She wanted to lose 70 pounds, and she insisted on doing it fast. I asked her how many times she tried that in the last 15 years, and then asked how that worked out for her in the past. All of a sudden, and this happens most of the time, she got defensive. (TIP: when you find yourself getting defensive, you're hiding or don't want to face the truth.)

Eventually, she agreed that all except the "last" time had failed. She had succeeded. She had lost the 70 pounds, but then she "blew" out her knee... and all the weight came back on. My response? Since when did gaining a massive 70 pounds become an inevitable side effect of injuring a knee? I asked why many who injure their knees don't put on the same weight?

She paused... then smiled, telling me, "I guess the 'last' time hadn't worked either."

So take the time right now and answer the simple question.

<u>WHY</u> do you want to lose weight?

Answering the previous three questions was a good place to start. (I'm talking about the exercise where I've asked you to list how your weight hurts you and others, and what was your single motivating factor for losing weight? If you DIDN'T take the time to do that exercise, you really should do it before going any further.)

"A diet that causes you to lose a lot of fat but leads to rebound, regain, and poor health DID NOT WORK"

Bottom line: if you're going to do this properly and permanently, you need to take the time and do this exercise thoroughly. You're going to NEED some serious, emotionally charged, and powerfully honest WHYs. When you do that, you will begin to have CLARITY.

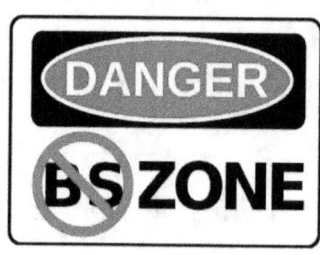

By the way, "CLARITY" <u>is needed, and is irrefutably necessary,</u> if success is to be had in ANY area of your life.

The Power of Belief

This is the last of the three dynamos that, if used and acted upon, will start breaking you free from your weight loss prison. Actually, if leveraged properly, they will break you out of any self-made prison. Social, financial, business, relationships, sporting endeavors, etc. All can be mastered by starting with these three dynamos.

What we think about most of the time is usually what we become. We tend to always move towards our most dominant thoughts. You may have heard it said, "Where focus goes, energy flows." This is so much more than a cute saying. It is a fact, and if you stop and think about it, you've experienced it many times.

The power of belief is apparent in our everyday lives, everywhere around us. When we see people over-come incredible odds and come out victorious, that's typically because they believed in themselves. Over time, our "outer" world becomes a reflection of our "inner" world. We can hide it temporarily, we can mask it for a while, but like trying to hold a balloon under water, it inevitably comes back to the surface.

Your thoughts (beliefs) are very powerful. They exert very strong influence over EVERYTHING in your life, especially your body. Your thoughts (beliefs) can make you happy or sad, can keep you awake at night, raise or lower your heart rate, make you afraid or bold, play havoc with your digestion, etc.

> "Success is not an accident.
> Sadly, failure is not an accident either"
> Brian Tracy

Your thoughts (beliefs) and the actions that are trig-gered by them run your whole life! Your beliefs are merely your interpretation of things and events, the stimuli that your brain digests every day. Beliefs held long enough are almost never questioned and are even held up as facts. All your actions or inactions are based on your beliefs that moving forward will either bring you some kind of pleasure or help you avoid pain. These processes dictate our every actions on a conscious or subconscious level. They dictate what we will do, what we contemplate, and what we immediately reject. Our long held beliefs even have control over how and what we think. They completely rule our lives, yet we rarely ever stop to consider their validity, their accurateness, and whether they're helping us or hurting us.

So please take the time to reconsider the source of your limiting beliefs while remembering that they are all based on your INTERPRETATIONS. It's high time you re-evaluate some of them so that they can better line up with the results you are looking for. This is your life. The question is: what kind of life are you looking for?

I won't spend too much time on this. I will say that without belief, nothing else matters. Of course, making the initial DECISION is still number one, and clarity is still number two. However, without belief, you won't follow through. You will self-sabotage. You will let something, somewhere derail your efforts. Justification will come very easily and often.

You MUST believe that you can be a healthy, slim you!

You MUST believe that you can do this.

This belief DOES NOT HAPPEN AUTOMATICALLY!

You must have a game plan. There has to be a strategy in place, a system, a path that you can follow. Your beliefs have to be worked on and DEVELOPED over time.

The last chapter of this book will review this area in a much deeper manner. By understanding how our conscious and subconscious minds work, we are able to set worthy goals and successfully achieve them.

A new you awaits!

However, before diving too deep into what ultimately affects our behaviours, there's some quick information I want to share that you can immediately put to good use. Let's start by looking at a few common dieting myths that many BELIEVE are facts. Keep in mind what we just talked about and how important beliefs are, as you may want to re-evaluate some of yours along the way.

Chapter Two:
Nine Myths That Are Destroying Your Weight Loss Goals

Not Looking Forward...

I was not looking forward to writing this chapter. I have no time for sensationalism and/or behaviour justifications. In today's world of excessive "political correctness" and ass kissing, it's getting harder and harder to separate the truth from the B.S. I understand that the truth is often unpleasant, unpopular, and draws unwarranted criticism, but for those who know me, I have always believed in "calling a spade, a spade."

After more than 13 years as the head coach, my job is not to "make friends" by telling you what you want to hear. People don't come to our club to get their ears tickled. They come here to lose weight, gain strength, increase their confidence, and get in shape.

Google the phrase "Top 5 Weight Loss Tricks" and see all the crap that comes up! Unfortunately, some people are indeed misinformed; they don't realize that what they have been reading IS utter crap. Don't get me wrong, there is some good stuff out there. I was pleasantly surprised at the "good and balanced" information that the National Institute of Diabetes and Digestive and Kidney Diseases had on their website, and there are plenty of others if you know where to look.

Here's a quick tip: if the web page loads slower than normal, if it's full of ads and other article headlines at the bottom and on the sides, it's most likely crap. Why? Because that page is there to MAKE MONEY, and the unfortunate truth is that you don't tend to make a lot of money by telling the truth. On the other hand, if you tell people what they want to hear, help alleviate their conscience, help them rationalise and justify their condition (however unhealthy), then most people will love you for it and buy your new trinket.

So, if you're looking for reliable, healthy, and useful weight loss information, you've come to the right place. However, you may not like what you find, and most likely you'll be forced to re-evaluate some of your preconceived beliefs.

Basic Rules

Before I begin, there are a few basic rules.

"Significant:" The use of this term is often abused and serves to mislead. It's easy to pick any myth or belief and say there is no "significant" research to prove it. One could say this about almost anything.

"Research:" The word "research" gets thrown around so much that it also becomes meaningless. What is "research" for one person is complete garbage to another. When it comes to calling it a "truth," I will always default to this: is the average person able to realistically replicate the results?

Duplicable and Long Term: This brings me to my sole determining success factor. When evaluating a weight loss strategy, are the results of using that strategy duplicable and long term? If the average person cannot realistically replicate the results then the strategy is of NO use to me or you. If the benefits are only short term, then this too is of <u>little</u> use to us. Remember, we want long term, permanent results.

Practicality: Some of the otherwise good information is so impractical and unrealistic in today's hectic life that it is rendered useless.

Expensive: If there is a cost, the strategy must be affordable to the average person.

There are several other factors to take into consideration, but it suffices to say that what really matters is if the strategy works in real life, is it duplicable, is it affordable, is it practical, is it healthy, and finally, are the results long term?

Now on to the nine myths...

> Even if you can't physically see the results in front of you, every single effort is changing your body from the inside out. Never forget that.

Myth #1: "A calorie is a calorie."

Yes, you could argue that a calorie is a unit of energy and that they are all the same, etc., etc.

Whoever is spouting that crap has never tried to lose weight.

When we say, "Not all calories are the same," we mean that not all calories **have the same effect on our bodies!**

Calories consumed from eating dark green vegetables will have a very different effect on your body then the same amount of calories consumed by drinking pop! The effect on your metabolism will be very different if you consume 300 calories from protein than from simple carbs. How soon after eating simple carbs are you hungry? Now compare that to eating a lean steak, assuming it has the same amount of calories.

As such, a calorie is NOT a calorie, and unless you educate yourself in this area, your weight loss endeavors will be a consistent "hit and miss" experience. Ultimately, poor caloric intake WILL leave you very frustrated and probably, well... FAT.

> "Success is the sum of small efforts, repeated day in and day out"

Myth #2: "You just don't have enough <u>willpower</u>."

This belief has harmed far too many people.

Many resign themselves to a life of frustration by thinking they cannot lose weight for a lack of discipline or willpower. How many times have we heard, "If only I had more willpower I could..."

Psychologists have long argued that "willpower" is a very complicated thing. Some say it's like a muscle, and the more you use it, the stronger it becomes. Others claim that they have located the specific place in the brain where willpower is found. Others claim it is some kind of spiritual force.

Personally, I'm not sure one way or the other. What I do know from research, personal experience, and observation is that **willpower is situational.** It is stronger in the mornings, stronger after eating, stronger after light exercise, stronger around certain people, etc. It is also weaker in the evenings, weaker in front of the TV, weaker with certain friends, weaker when we are tired, etc.

If you are honest with yourself, I'm sure you agree that "willpower" is undependable. It's often weak, and it's usually lacking when you need it the most. It fluctuates wildly. For many, it's just a figment of their imagination and has proven to be absolutely UNDE-PENDABLE.

Willpower need only be used to help control our thoughts and internal conversations. Manage to change your thinking patterns and almost all else will fall into place. Willpower should NOT be "the" determining factor regarding your weight loss progress. If it is, the minute life throws you a curve ball and you get distracted, all progress will cease and you will start moving backward. This is what we refer to as "yo-yo" dieting.

> "It's not what you are that is holding you back. It's what you think you are not."

The real, unfortunate result when one believes that a lack of willpower is what stands in their way is the serious ramifications it presents in so many OTHER areas of their life. Many erroneously conclude that if they lack willpower in one area, they must lack it in others. With this belief firmly imbedded in their minds (consciously or subconsciously), many other areas suffer and the "compounding effect" can be disastrous.

What you end up with is a low self-image, and that my friend affects EVERYTHING! That means family, financial, social, business, sports, and of course, your health and your happiness. These are all negatively affected by a low self-image. Your self-image is part of your psychology, and psychology is by far THE most important determinant of success in ALL areas of your life. I've always said, "Life is won or lost in your mind FIRST."

Simply put, if your "thinking" is flawed regarding weight loss, then your chances of success are slim.

Myth #3: "It's simple, eat less and move more."

I would love to spar with whoever says this! I would deck them with a lead hook, and after landing a few blows, I would just say, "It's simple, just move more!"

Even though technically one can't argue with the statement, when it comes to <u>sustained</u> weight loss, it's just NEVER that simple. Not even close. You may get away with it (it will work) for the first few pounds, but then your body has several surprises waiting for you.

At the risk of oversimplifying things this is what happens with this piece of wisdom.

When you eat less, your metabolism starts to slow down. You have much less energy, and don't feel like moving at all, much less more. Your motivation goes down the crapper, and without it you don't feel like doing anything except watch Netflix and eat crappy food. Your hunger drives you nuts, and all you think about is food. Reduce your food intake enough for extended period of time, and your body will start cannibalising its own muscles. Since it's your muscles that burn calories, your metabolism slows down even more. This starts affecting EVERYTHING else in your life. The "compounding effects" start to take their toll. **It only gets worse from here.**

Move more? Try doing that with the above conditions! Not to mention moving more will burn additional calories and lower your blood sugar levels that much more. Then the glucose stored in your liver will be the next thing to go. Then surprise... you're cranky, totally un-motivated (more likely depressed), have no energy, starving, and wanting to eat everything in the house. At this point, "moving more" will substantially increase or worsen all your symptoms.

I wish it was that simple, but the reality of successfully losing weight permanently is much more complex. I didn't say "impossible." I said "complex"

It is doable, and yes, <u>YOU can do it.</u>

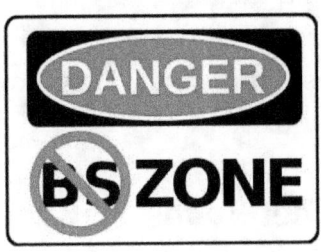

"Eat less and move more" only works for the first few pounds when you start a "diet." After that, you'd better have some good information, tools, and a strategic game plan. Let's not repeat what has never worked before. **There is a way, and it's not that hard!**

(Assuming you are using the right tools and strategies, of course.)

Myth #4: "Such and such diet really works, I lost 30 pounds..."

Listen, I won't spend much time on this one.

"Diets" DO NOT WORK.

Period.

End of discussion.

Low calorie diets, low fat diets, no carb diets, high fiber diets, cleansing diets, single food diets, fasting diets, timing diets, food combining diets, vegetarian diets, high protein diets...

Seriously, this is not a game. They do not work. Never have, never will.

Myth #5: "Diet foods will help you lose weight and keep it off."

This is a particularly dangerous one because it often leads unsuspecting people to develop various food addictions.

Out of all the crazy advice and beliefs out there, this one can lead to very poor health and virtually GUARANTEES that you will stay fat.
Take diet pop. "But it only has five calories!" Perhaps, but now you drink three instead of one. Not to mention, it is full of crap that is not healthy for you. The "fake sugars" are chemicals that wreak havoc on your body and mind. You still get an insulin spike that

drives and packs more fat into your fat cells... Your poor liver has to work overtime cleaning all this crap out of your system. Worst of all, many of these "diet products" are ADICTIVE!

Your body was NOT designed to process POP. It was designed to benefit from WATER. Notice I didn't say "process" water. There's nothing to process. Instead of slowing everything down and using up energy to process all kinds of crap and desperately trying to excrete it out of your system, when you drink good old water, your body saves a lot of otherwise wasted energy.

It gets to the point that many people simply DON'T drink water! "Water is too bland, it's tasteless..." It's called borderline addiction! If you want some taste, just add some lemon, lime, or even cucumbers. It actually tastes good without damaging your body.

Listen, junk foods are "designed" to be fun, to taste good, to make you "feel" great, <u>and to be addictive.</u>

Ever wonder why you have a hard time changing your diet? The food industry literally spends millions on research to find out the combination of ingredients, additives, and preservatives that keep you buying more and more. They want this to continue forever. These foods are designed to trigger the pleasure center of the brain. Ever wonder why you often feel "good" right after eating crap? (At least until your conscience kicks in.) No one in their right mind enjoys being obese or having chronic diseases, but many find it almost impossible to change their eating habits.

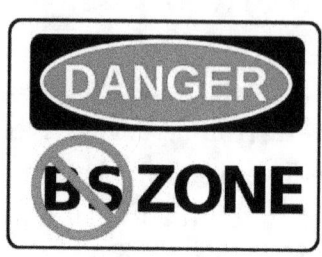

Bottom line: whenever you see the following words, you know that crap is going to be bad for you in many known and unknown ways. That includes being addictive by targeting the pleasure centers in your brain. So remember, you should be avoiding things that claim to be:

- Low Fat
- Sugar Free
- Fat Free
- Processed
- Gluten Free
- Instant
- No Sugar Added

If you see these things... RUN!

Think I'm exaggerating? Research "MSG," what it does to you, how it works on your brain, and why they put it in so many processed foods!

Myth #6: "Have you tried product (X)? I've already lost 10 pounds..."

There's really not much to say here. We all know times when we've been foolish and thrown away our hard earned money on some "easy way out" scam. The sad thing about it is that we weren't even upset when it didn't work because "we knew." Hah! To make things worse, some people will repeatedly try these quack job products, and the worst of us even actively look for these short cuts and magic pills and potions! In the last 13 years, do you know how many times I've heard, "I've tried EVERYTHING."

My answer is always, "Great, now maybe we can get serious."

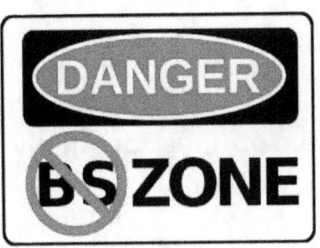

Let's be very clear. There are no miracle cures. There are no secret potions. Not even liposuction or gastral bypass surgery! I don't care what the movie stars do. Look at the risks. Look at the long term success rate. Finally, look at it this way. If you try to take short cuts on something as important as your health, then you will try to take short cuts EVERYWHERE you can. Boy, that will lead to a full and rich life. **NOT!** So do yourself a favour, and cut the foolishness.

> "Nothing tastes as good as thin FEELS."

Myth #7: "You should always have a cheat day."

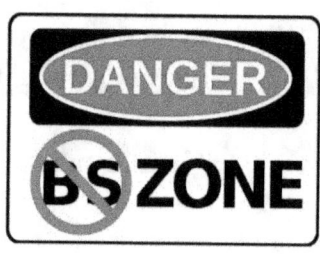

***WARNING** If your blood sugar levels are low, if you've had a bad day, if it's just not your fault... blah, blah, blah! You most definitely do not want to read this right now.

Don't say I didn't warn you. Here goes. If 70% of the population has a weight problem and most of them have "tried EVERYTHING..." And if 90% never succeed, only "yo-yo," and put on a little more weight every year all while using "cheat days," what makes you think you will have different results?

People complain that it's not their fault because they're "addicted" to chocolate, addicted to pop, addicted to chips, sweets, etc. I agree, but seriously, would you tell a recovering alcoholic that it's alright to have a "cheat" day? How about a recovering cocaine addict? See the foolishness in this thinking?

Not so fast. Before you mentally start arguing with me, have you or have you not ever said that you were addicted to ____? No? Then why don't you just STOP? You can't have it both ways. What are we, a bunch of little children? Seriously.

People repeatedly underestimate the addictive power of refined foods.

Let me ask you this:

How do they make cocaine?

How do they make heroin?

Now consider this:
How do they make sugar?

How do they make white flour?

COCAINE: They use COCA leaves and refine them into a nice fine powder...

HEROIN: They use POPPY plants and refine them into a nice fine powder…

SUGAR: They use the sugar canes and refine them into a nice fine powder…

FLOUR: They use various plants, grains, etc. and refine them into a nice fine powder…

See a trend?

YES, I agree with cheat days. The research backs it up. They are useful. They have several specific purposes. They definitely have their strategic place in a well-designed weight loss strategy. However, not all cheat days are created equal!

Do you even know why you should have cheat days? It's definitely not so you could indulge in your addictions or reward yourself for good behavior (following your diet). There are several purposes, but here's one of them. In a successful program they are strategically used to "jump start" your metabolism and "rev-up" your calorie burning engine. Not to mention, a bad cheat day can damage and negate a week's worth of disciplined eating! If that cheat day happens to be on a Friday, boy you have big problems. Friday quickly turns into, "I'll start again on Monday," and then soon that's followed by, "I've tried everything!"

I'll stop here. I'm sure I've irritated enough people.

Never forget…

"You are 100% responsible."

(By the way, if you're thinking "I can't do this without cheat days" then you are probably doing several things wrong.)

Myth #8: "Cardio is best for weight loss."

Yes, cardio is good. It does absolute wonders for your circulatory system. It is fantastic for your heart and lungs. Movement is also great for your lymphatic system. It helps your body transport nutrients and flushes all kinds of debris. We are also just beginning to scratch the surface of what it does to our minds. But it simply isn't the end all, be all for weight loss. Remember, it is your muscles that burn calories, and cardio is far from being the best type of exercise for toning, strengthening, and maintaining (building) strong muscles. So there lies the problem.

People tend to go overboard with cardio. They do too much. At first, the weight tends to come off quickly, and as a result, people are encouraged. If a little works, more must be better, right? These are the two things that I've seen through the years that end up causing "cardio" to be counter-productive:

#1 - The first problem is that it takes too much time out of a typical week. At first this is not a problem because the weight is coming off and all is well, but soon, your body adapts to the new workload and the same workouts are no longer resulting in reduced weight. So what do people do? They do more cardio. Result... weight loss resumes for a while longer. Then it soon stops again. Actually, now you are starting to get "repetitive use" injuries and/or irritations. You're feeling a bit run-down and find yourself susceptible to colds and the flu as your immune system starts to weaken. Another problem with "more cardio" strategy is that you soon find yourself with NO life as you're always spending time doing cardio. It only takes a weekend or two of fun with the friends, and out goes all the best of intentions as you rationalise that there's more to life than just exercising all the time.

#2 - The other problem with more and more cardio is that it generally cannibalises your muscles. These are the very muscles you need to keep the metabolism furnace burning. Remember, muscles are what burns calories. Quickly Google pictures of sprinters (short, high intensity training) and long distance runners (long cardio). See the incredible difference? Besides, it's not just about "losing weight," it's about health and being fit (and looking good). No man ever watched a women go by and commented, "Look at that hot 138.5 pound woman." It's not how much you weigh, it's HOW you look!

Myth #9: "Fat is bad."

I'll keep this one very short. There are good fats and not so good fats. I personally believe you almost can't have too much quality fish and coconut oil. (I say almost because there are always people who will...)

Do a quick Google search of all the benefits of coconut oil! You will be very surprised. If your brain starts asking, "How can fat be good when you're trying to lose fat?" then it's time to ignore your brain. Tell it to be quiet. Here's an oversimplification. When your body is getting plenty of good quality healthy oils, it will feel free to shed fat. If your body is starving for good quality oils, it will tend to hang on to as much fat as possible.

Remember the Myths

There you have it, nine "myths" that countless people struggle with when they're looking for successful weight loss. Unfortunately, there are MANY more damaging beliefs out there that make it confusing for the average person to lose weight permanently. It is important that your sources of information are truly reliable to help avoid these types of myths.

> "What fits your busy schedule better, exercise one hour a day or being dead 24 hours a day?

In the next chapter, we will touch on an area that many really struggle with: food CRAVINGS. Just getting control in this area alone would solve the extra weight issue for a good percentage of the population. The biggest problem I find in this area is a complete misunderstanding of what cravings are, how they work, and how to modify or overcome them entirely. I've had to simplify things considerably in the following chapter, as several books could be written on this subject alone. I've purposefully kept things simple and very practical to help foster a basic understanding and encourage success. Now let's move on to chapter three!

Chapter Three:
Food Cravings, and Nine Ways to Stop Them Dead Every Time

Willpower?

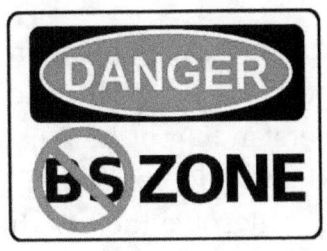

Let's be very clear on one thing. If your strategy for overcoming food cravings is to use willpower, you are "dead in the water," you are "toast." Seriously, how has that worked out for you in the past? (I know I keep asking you this.) It doesn't matter if "this time" you have "more discipline, more willpower, and it's going to work..." No, it won't. It never has, and it never will. Willpower is a very deceptive train of thought. Willpower is extremely SITUATIONAL. Monday morning, you have massive willpower. Friday evening in front of the TV, not so much!

The bottom line: if your strategy for overcoming food cravings is willpower, you are doomed to fail. At the very least, you will be leading a life of NEVER

ENDING struggle. Why not take a bit of time and learn how to "fix" this permanently?

> Life only truly begins once we start accepting 100% full responsibility for our lives.

Before we begin... I'd like to mention again that for a small percentage of weight challenged people, acquiring a good understanding of how habits are formed, how they work, and how to modify them is all they need to permanently solve their "extra" weight challenge. So even though I've greatly simplified this chapter, don't underestimate the absolutely incredible power of habits.

What Are Food Cravings?

Unfortunately, we've all experienced these more than once. There comes an almost irresistible urge to eat, and it's usually very specific foods (crap). Some of the more popular cravings are chocolate, ice cream, chips, etc. These can hardly be called foods. They're more like chemical soups that trigger very specific and dependable physical and mental reactions.

To make things worse, repeated often enough (less than most think), the memory center of the brain becomes involved. Before you know it, you're "hooked." It has now become a powerful habit that many NEVER break free from.

Every time the junk food habit is repeated, it becomes more ingrained as more neural pathways are developed and strengthened between the triggers and the accompanying responses. Yes, it becomes an addiction.

What makes this worse is that, for the most part, these "foods" are SPECIFICALLY DESIGNED to trigger and develop these addictive responses. It's called "business."

Ideally, one is best to avoid developing these habits, but if you're reading this book, the odds are it is too late. You may have already developed several of these.

> "We become what we repeatedly do."
> Sean Covev

It's All in Your Head, Really

(Ok, maybe not all of it, haha.)

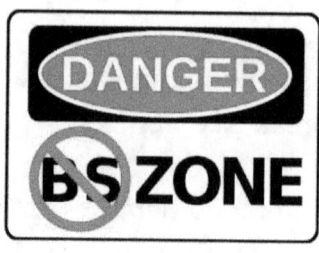

You need to understand that it's not "in your genes." Yes some are more susceptible than others, but you still can't just dismiss responsibility as if it were completely out of your control. It is fully and completely in your control. As with most everything else, you are 100% responsible, and the minute you decide that you're not, you are "toast." It's really very simple. The minute you start playing the "victim" card is the minute you start giving away all your power.

With the knowledge you are accumulating from these pages, you will have all the tools and strategies necessary for complete success.

Mix that with some honest perseverance and willingness to notice what's working and what's not, followed by slight adjustments, and you will absolutely succeed.

The very first step is to recognize and admit that these cravings are a problem. The next step is developing a few simple but effective strategies for dealing with or preventing them. Finally, with a bit of work and a few strategies for dismantling them, we will successfully reduce or even eliminate their effects on us.

Life is Easier with "Systems"

When we say, "It's all in your head," what we mean is it begins and ends in your brain.

This is another reason why, without proper knowledge and a few strategies, many people never achieve victory in this area. Our bodies AND our brains are designed to run on "systems." There is a "system" for just about everything we do and even the way we think. This includes our thought processes, our feelings, our interpretations, how we see the world, how we see ourselves, and so on.

The line between "systems," "habits," and "processes" are blurry, and sometimes I will interchange the terms.

Very Basic Mechanics

Let's look at a typical example. Assume you work at a computer in an office or at home. There are usually several tasks that are repetitive, meaning you do them either daily or weekly. Some of these tasks you hate (stress). Maybe you tend to put them off until there's a deadline of some sorts, which adds "pressure" (stress). When these tasks should be getting finished, you start looking for distractions. (This is often done at the subconscious level.) Eventually, it has to be done. At the highest point of stress, a craving (escape) is triggered, and we know exactly where the "stash" is or the person to go see. Before you know it, the whole chocolate bar is gone, a rush of serotonin (happy chemical) washes through the "reward center" of your brain, and your memory center connects the chocolate bar with this pleasant sensation. The next time a similar stress is experienced or even perceived (trigger), the craving for chocolate will hit you even harder. New neural connections and pathways are being formed and strengthened more and more every time until you are effectively "addicted."

This is the same process whether it's a financial stress, marital stress, or stress with a boss or co-worker, etc.

Succumbing to your cravings becomes easier. Then we beat ourselves up mentally, which just reinforces and strengthens all the neural connections!

It can escalate to the point where if this trigger happens at roughly the same time every day, the process will start WITHOUT the trigger. In other words, the time itself will be the trigger.

Maybe It's Just a Bad Habit?

Sometimes there is no need for a stressor or a trigger. Often it is just a habit. Friday night... watch a movie... unwind... eat crap. It may have initially started with stress, but it is simply habit at this point regardless of stress. We can't even watch a movie without 800 calories of garbage. The patterns or "systems" are well set, and the neural connections are like steel cables.

It has absolutely nothing to do with will power.

Triggers, We All Have Them!

We must start recognizing or even anticipating our triggers. Acknowledging them, we can start putting together proper and effective strategies that will enable us to get past these triggers and their accompanying cravings (binges).

It all starts with "mindfulness," the process of living in the "now." More specifically, noticing what is happening when we are being triggered, the "what" of our triggers. What exactly is causing these triggers? Is it habit? Stress? Boredom? Perhaps it's feeling lonely, feeling that you "deserve" something, or even feeling afraid? Start living in the "now" more often. Start noticing things in "real time." With mindfulness, you will quickly notice and come to realize all of your triggers and what causes them. Once you know your triggers, we are "off to the races," and only then can we start making real progress. This should only take two or three weeks at the most.

A side note...

Keep in mind that when we fully accept personal responsibility, understand how cravings work, and implement proper strategies to avoid the binges, we may NEVER need to diet! Just eliminating the binges will suffice. Add regular exercising, and big things will begin to happen. Not just weight loss, but your health will dramatically improve, your self-image and confidence will go through the roof. That is, if you leverage what you've learnt and the new skills you've acquired to other areas of your life... Get the picture?

Continuing with Mindfulness

Now that we've identified "what" causes our triggers and our cravings, the next step is to notice <u>how we respond</u>. Notice your food choices. Are they spicy? Are they sweet or fatty? Often, it's a combination.

Have you noticed that you are not really hungry!? Assuming you are eating normally and haven't gone an unusual amount of time without food, this is **not** your body's way of telling you that it's hungry. It is purely mental, emotional, and habitual.

> "You control and develop your habits, or your habits control and develop you!"

Once you've practiced mindfulness for a few weeks, you will see the same patterns. It's now time to strategize and overcome them.

Strategizing

At this point, I am assuming that you understand how cravings work and how they are triggered. I'm assuming you've spent at least two or three weeks practicing mindfulness, and you grasp what your triggers are, when they usually happen, and how you normally respond. Without taking the time to properly lay this foundation, trying to implement these strategies may prove frustrating.

So again, one last time:

- #1 - There is a "trigger." It could be a stressor, a time, place, event, person, etc.
- #2 - That is followed by your "response." This response is often the same, like grabbing for a chocolate bar.

#3 - The resulting hormonal and chemical reactions in the brain produces a sense of pleasure...

#4 - The brain "wires" these three together and remembers them. (Neurons that fire together, wire together.)

#5 - Through time and repetition, the neural connections grow stronger and stronger.

Start over? I don't think so.

Now we could start over, we could totally undo the bad habit. It is doable. It will take a knowledgeable therapist, skilled in this area, and it will take time and money. Lots of it. First, we will have to retrain our brain to interpret the trigger differently. Then we must start working on forming new neuro-associations, and finally link them to new responses. Doable, yes. Practical, not so much.

There is a much easier way, a much cheaper way, a much quicker way.

Start with the trigger. Chances are that this trigger will be around for a while. Since we can't always avoid it, let's use it to our advantage instead. While we are at it, why not use the existing neural connections? Why not just change our final response? The formula is simple:

#1 - Use existing trigger
#2 - Use existing neural pathways
#3 - Change our final response

(Yes, this is a gross oversimplification.)

Strategy #1: Get up immediately and do something.

(Preferably something physically challenging.)

Take the time to experiment here and find out what works best for you. Also, what is most practical? Often, the single best action is to **quickly** remove yourself from the current environment, such as taking a short, brisk walk. Unfortunately, this may be impossible if you are at work. In that case, perhaps doing 30 or 50 slow, deep squats and ending with 20 fast ones would be better? Maybe quickly going up three flights of stairs and come back down.

The key here is to spot the trigger and **quickly** change the usual response. An aggressive physical response (some type of exercise) is best because it does a couple things for you:

#1 - It may take you physically out of the triggering environment.

#2 - It will force you to change your focus, which is in itself priceless.

Exercising will raise your heart rate and your breathing rate. Both have their own list of physical, emotional, and mental benefits. More importantly, your brain will start to modify your neural pathways and connections between the triggers and "fitness."

Neural pathways tend to be stronger when there is some kind of "physicality" and/or "emotions" attached to them. At the very least, you will burn some calories.

The bottom line: don't delay. Act as soon as you feel the trigger coming. This helps your brain begin modifying your neural connections and pathways between the trigger and the new behavior. If the trigger or response changes are significant enough, the old habits will slowly start to degrade and lose their strength. This all takes time and repetition. There are no short cuts.

One last thing… if you try to "reason" or debate in your mind whether you really need to do those squats or go up three flights of stairs, you will not get the benefits. In fact, you will probably succumb to the temptation. Do not "play" with it in your head. Immediately get up and …

Strategy #2: Plan ahead with almonds and nuts.

Raw almonds, raw sunflower seeds, plenty of large coconut chips, and dried banana chips all mixed together would be my second weapon. These should all be purchased at a health food store with no sugar, salt, or MSG. This is a powerful weapon against triggered cravings for several reasons. (The banana chips may be coated with sugar? No big deal.)

They don't spoil easily, and they don't need to be refrigerated. The almonds and sunflower seeds slow down your digestion, help to stabilize your blood sugar levels, and help keep you feeling full. The coconut chips are high in healthy "good" fats that also slow down digestion. This helps you feel satisfied for longer. The dried bananas give it all a sweet touch (taste). Lastly, the myriad of health benefits of almonds, coconut, and sunflower seeds are absolutely amazing.

With repetition and time, your brain will associate the trigger with the healthy snack, and the problem will be well on its way to being solved, effectively rewired. (By the way, this process can be sped up with positive affirmations, visualisation, etc.)

Extra bonus! It will help if, after being triggered, you ate this while walking, going to a window looking outside, listening to music, etc. There are many other options. Do whatever is appropriate under the circumstances.

Strategy #3: Plan ahead with protein.

If the cravings are not necessarily "triggered" by stress or some strong emotional reasons, but more of a physical hunger, a simple solution can be as easy as increasing your protein intake. Lean meats take longer to digest and help keep you feeling satisfied much longer than carbs, especially simple carbs. Protein meals help stabilize blood sugar levels and will help if you are prone to "sugar mood swings" followed by cravings.

Be careful. Often, when my students start their process, they are all psyched-up. They've cut out this and that, and they've decided to not eat meat anymore, etc. My response is always the same. "Will this dietary plan be forever?"

At this point, they explain that this will only be while they're dieting and losing weight... that is a bad idea. It's not the fact that they've cut out meat, but that they are using <u>non-sustainable</u> methods. If you plan on eating meat after you reach your target weight, you should continue eating meat while slowly reducing your body weight. Otherwise, your weight loss will not be sustainable, and all the work will have been for nothing.

Bottom line is that you should know your triggers and when they will most likely occur. Also, be aware of possible extended times with no food intake. A little planning with meats will go a long ways to prevent, or at least significantly decrease, your cravings. Incorporating high protein meals when you expect a lengthy part of the day with no food and/or higher than normal temptations will help you get through them successfully.

Strategy #4: Short term planning with fiber.

What do you do when it's apparent that you're about to find yourself in a situation where triggers are likely and your odds of success feel slim to none? Better yet, what about the times when you KNOW you're about to be BAD. For those occasions, I have a quick fix.

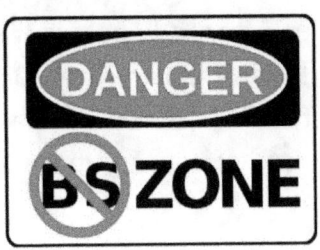

I have personally used this trick very effectively because it works. It becomes a problem when a person starts to use this trick as a STRATEGY in itself to get away with bad dietary habits, or even worse as a way to somehow get around cravings and addictions. Using this trick whenever "triggered" totally defeats what you are trying to do. You are working on "rewiring" your neural connections or pathways between the triggers and the reward. To maintain the same reward and hope to mitigate the damages is almost pointless. This should not be used when trying to modify behaviour. It is strictly to be used sparingly, when you're about to be "bad."

Here it is. A quick large, **full** glass of water mixed with psyllium husk fiber. This does the trick the majority of the time. It keeps you satisfied. It's easy to take. It's instant. It does wonders for your colon and your cholesterol levels. It's inexpensive. There's no cooking, etc.

Remember, I said "instant." I'm not kidding. Once you put the psyllium fiber in the cup and mix it, you have about 10 to 15 seconds before it starts to turn to gel! Then, swallowing starts to become "awkward." Also, you must drink plenty of water. This is important. The desired effects are felt within a few short minutes.

One last time: drink plenty of water.

Strategy #5: Review and focus on your physical goals.

Taking a few minutes to re-write your goals, or better yet work on your "vision board," is a great way to re-direct your focus. Like Tony Robins says, "Where focus goes, energy flows." I know it sounds a bit corny, but hey, "As a man thinketh, so is he." You may want to start keeping a binder with several (many) various pics of athletic people you aspire to emulate. If you are writing your goals out, you may want to say them out loud. Even better, add some emotions to it all while visualising your end results or your desired outcomes.

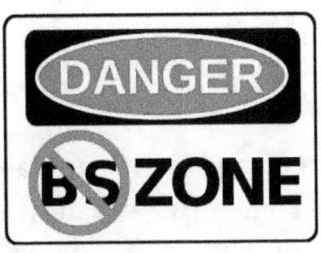

Do NOT underestimate the power of "focus." Our outer world is indeed a reflection of our inner world. The quality of your thinking determines the quality of your life to a great extent. When we think about crap, we feel like crap. There is no denying it. The same is true when we think about good stuff (like a forthcoming sunny vacation). We feel great in no time. Like I've said earlier in the book, "Life is won or lost in your mind first." So when tempted or when cravings hit, a few minutes spent emotionally focused on your goals and what you want out of life will often be all you need to tie you over.

This strategy can be used by itself, but for even better results, it can be combined with others to increase their effectiveness.

Strategy #6: Sometimes it's as simple as leaving.

That's right. Are you tempted? Do you know "it" is coming? Sometimes the best and most effective action to take is to simply leave! You may not feel like it. It may be a pain in the ass, but what is the alternative? Are you serious or not?

Let's say you're at work. At such and such time, a specific person comes by. When you interact with them, the odds of getting "triggered" are raised exponentially. Just leave before they arrive. This strategy can be used effectively in many different scenarios. Most often, these involve people. Be wise. Be healthy.

Strategy #7: Reduce the stress.

People make this one much harder than it really needs to be. Going back to the beginning of this chapter, <u>strategy #7 can only work if you accept 100%</u> <u>personal responsibility for your life.</u>

You need to understand that stress is caused on the "inside." Stress is internal and not external. Stress is a result of the INTERPRETATION and the meaning you are giving the situation or "thing" and nothing else. Understanding this will go a long way in making life much more enjoyable.

Let's look at a couple quick examples. I say "quick" because people either see how simple this stress thing really is, or they fight it and play the "victim card" while giving away all their power.

Example #1.
My wife is 45 minutes late picking me up.

"She's supposed to pick me up. She knows I hate waiting. Why does she do that? She knows I'm out here, and that it's raining. She's doing this on purpose. She knows I don't even have a coat on.... Why does she cause me so much stress...?"

Example #2.
My wife is 45 minutes late picking me up.

"I wonder what's going on? I hope everything is okay. I wonder if she's stuck in traffic? I hope she's okay..."

Which of the two examples will leave me upset, angry, and all stressed out, and which one will leave me feeling in a more peaceful and loving state?

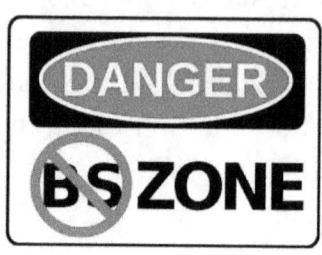

Stress is always caused by the interpretation or the meanings we give to things and/or events. This is why some people are destroyed by the very same things that help others grow and become more than previously seemed possible. This is why two people can see and explain the same things differently. Is the glass half empty or half full? Seriously. It really is that simple, but only if you accept 100% responsibility.

Does someone make you feel inferior? Why? Only you can allow yourself to feel that; it's your interpretations not their actions. It's like people who carry grudges (baggage) all their lives. "You don't know what this person did to me..." Meanwhile the other person is clueless or has long forgotten. Stress is internal. There will be some that get irritated (stressed) at me while reading this. I don't even know who they are! Haha! Again, the stress they are feeling is because of their interpretations. Stress is internal, not external.

Bottom line: you may want to re-interpret the meanings you attribute to things and/or hold towards some people or events in your life that are causing you stress. Start with the simple ones, and then work your way up to the more challenging ones. It takes time and mindfulness, but it will help dramatically.

Strategy #8: Sleep.

This is a simple one. Are you getting enough sleep? Recent research has shown that a few sleepless nights is all it takes to drop your "leptin" hormone levels by about 18% while boosting your "ghrelin" levels. Leptin is the hormone that signals satiety; in other words, it tells you that you've had enough. Obviously when these are low, temptations are more frequent and can be more intense. Ghrelin is a hormone that triggers appetite. You may have noticed these effects after a "rough" few days with less or low quality sleep or even when you work the night shift. It also can happen when you change time zones.

Just like brain studies, "sleep" is another area with new findings coming out almost daily. There too, we are only now starting to learn and understand what's involved and the corresponding effects.

Help avoid needless cravings. Get enough sleep.

Strategy #9: Brush your teeth. What?

Another simple one. This strategy works well for a surprising amount of people. When a craving hits, get up and give your teeth a good brushing. Preferably with a clean, minty toothpaste.

Why does this work? Maybe it's because you had to leave the environment? Maybe it's because you had to get up, walk to another room, and brush (physical activity)? Maybe it's because it plays with your taste buds? Perhaps it's as simple as having your mouth feel and taste clean and minty, so you'd like to leave it like that.

Most likely, it works well because of all the small and synergistically effective strategies described above.

But I Still Get Cravings!

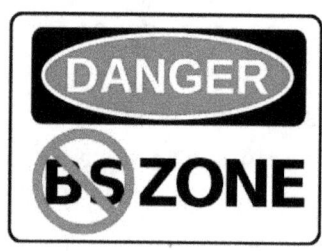

The title of this section is "Nine Ways to <u>Stop</u>...", but **YOU** have to stop them. **YOU** have to do something. It doesn't say, "Nine Ways to Make Them Disappear." Listen, if you are in your late 40s, you've been building and strengthening these habitual neural connections for the last 20-plus YEARS. Did you think they would just disappear? Are you serious and want permanent results, or are you just looking for a temporary quick fix? Do you plan on failing again and starting all over in a few months? I hope not. I'm assuming that this time you want to learn and do everything the correct and permanent way. Enough is enough, don't you think?

Learn to do this properly and you can build the life of your dreams. Why? Because the process of changing neural connections and pathways is the same in every area of your life, including finances, relationships, etc.

You can form new empowering habits, new neural connections, that will move you closer to your goals in a much faster and productive way. Think about the two or three areas in your life where limiting beliefs have held you back and prevented you from living the life you originally planned back when you were in your early twenties.

To your complete success!

Chapter Four:
Resetting Your
Body Weight Set Point

Can you relate to this?

When we're young, we have dreams of what our lives will look like. It usually involves being healthy, wealthy, successful, marrying a great spouse, and living in a nice place. Then life gets in the way and ultimately takes over. We lose control, and our dreams slowly and gradually get postponed. After repeated failed attempts, we slowly "settle" to living a life far below our original expectations. It can be a painful existence, especially KNOWING we are so much better and more capable than that!

Over time, even the best of us become frustrated.

You may be feeling like that now: completely frustrated with your results or lack thereof in one or more areas of your life. It's not entirely your fault. You were not trained in HOW to achieve your dreams, and today there is far too much conflicting information out there! You're not alone. The key is what actions you take today. How will you make the most of your second chance?

Are you "sick and tired of being sick and tired?"

Don't settle for a life you never really wanted.

Adjusting Your Thermostat.

Before we dive into this most revealing topic, we need to modify one little thing. The words "set point." It should be called a "settling point" instead. "Set point" infers an unchanging permanent point. However, we know that's not true because we've all watched our weight fluctuate. You're likely thinking, "Yes, I've lost weight before, but I always put it all back on and more." There you go! You increased your set point. Haha (okay, it's not funny). The truth is, unlike many others our mental and bodyweight "set points", are more aptly called "settling points." More on this later.

What Is a "Set Point?"

Many initially assume they're not familiar with set points. A set point is a **condition** that your body is comfortable in, but it's much more than that. Here are just a few examples of the countless set points our body maintains on a constant basis:

- Your body temperature
- Your blood pressure

- Your body's PH levels (acidity)
- Your blood's PH levels (acidity)
- Your actual blood levels
- How much water you hold
- Your oxygen levels
- Your blood glucose
- Cellular fluid balance
- Sodium levels
- Calcium levels
- Hormone levels

In the short term, your metabolism and how many calories you burn try to stay within a "set point." This extends to your body fat levels and even how much "muscle" you carry.

There are also complete "system" set points. Your mind and belief systems have their own set points (self-image)! Your body is designed to stay in a state of equilibrium. This balance is a survival mechanism. When things are in equilibrium, the body uses much less energy to keep things humming along smoothly.

Let's take a look at some quick examples of "set points."

First, there's the temperature set point in your house and how your thermostat keeps it perfectly in the range that you set it at.

A thermostat is a servomechanism, a small piece of technology that can be given a "goal" and does what it can to reach this goal and stay there. The one in my house operates like this:

It takes the current temperature in the house. Next, it compares it to what it has been programmed to keep the house at. In this case, let's say I set it for 70° F. Let's assume I just came home, and while I was away, the thermostat was set at 68° F. Obviously, the thermostat senses that it needs to bring up the temperature by two degrees. It sends a signal to the furnace to light up and start the heating process. In several minutes, it senses that the temperature has reached 70° F, so it sends a signal for the furnace to shut off. From that point, the house slowly but gradually starts to cool off. When the temperature in the house reaches around 69° F, the thermostat sends another signal for the furnace to kick on again. Minutes later, it is 70° F in the house. Once again, the thermostat sends another signal for the furnace to shut off. This process continues uninterrupted until I give it a new order, a new setting.

Example of a mental or a self-image set point:

This is especially apparent in sales people. Their income fluctuates up and down within predictable limits, and very rarely does it fluctuate too far out of that range. When it does, it is only short term. If a salesman sees himself as an earner that makes $60,000/annually ($5,000/month), his performance will generally stay around there for years and maybe even for life unless his psychology changes. Even in "hard times," he will maintain that income range, just a little higher and a little lower. When he hits a bad streak and his income drops, he works longer hours, he makes sure he is productive, he brushes up on his skills, makes more calls, and basically does whatever a salesman on a $60,000 salary needs to do to earn that figure. After all, he's a $60,000 producer! That's who he is. When his income starts getting comfortably over $5,000 per month, whether he knows it or not, he starts to self-sabotage. After all, things are going well, and he "deserves" a bit of time off! There's more to life than just work, right? He makes less calls, starts to procrastinate, becomes less efficient... You see his self-image does NOT see him as a $75,000/annual earner. Actually, he starts to feel uncomfortable. Deep down, his subconscious says that he doesn't deserve this lifestyle, that maybe he is overcharging his customers, etc. Although most would not admit it, nor even be aware of what's happening, their self-image, their subconscious, always finds subtle ways to ever so slightly mess things up. In no time, sales start to dry up, and his income starts to drop. Once it reaches below his self-image concept, his self-talk starts to change. He starts telling himself that he needs to pull his shit together, that he's better than this, that he's done it before and can do it again, that his family depends on him, etc. He becomes more efficient, starts making more calls, and so on. The result? His income starts to increase and falls back into his self-image range. It doesn't matter if the economy gets bad (he just works harder) or if the economy gets really good (he unknowingly self-sabotages even more). Ultimately, his self-image set point will keep him in the $60,000 salary range.

There are many other examples we could use. These are often called "comfort-zones."

What Is a Body Weight Set Point?

Your body weight set point, or "settling" point, operates much the same way. It is a range in which your body fat levels or percentage are the most easily maintained and both your body and **MIND** are comfortable with. (The MIND part is covered in the next section.) This body weight is successfully maintained, plus or minus a few pounds, on a daily and weekly basis. Granted, it has hundreds of inputs to monitor and is obviously much more complicated, but the principles are all the same. It receives orders to maintain the fat percentage in a certain range, and it does just that.

Now let's look at what happens when we mess with the system...

Eating too many calories, or at least more than usual...

Assuming you are currently within your set point, whenever you eat too many calories, your body has several mechanisms that start kicking in to get rid of these extra calories in an effort to keep your weight within your set point. Examples:

- Your appetite decreases below normal.
- Your metabolism (your engine) will start to "rev-up" and burn more.
- Your resting heart rate will want to increase above normal.
- Your breathing will want to increase above normal.
- You may start getting a bit "fidgety."
- Your attitude generally turns more positive.
- Your thinking changes more towards "doing" things.
- Depending if you just binged, you may even start sweating.

These and many other changes start immediately, and their purpose is to burn off the extra calories so that you don't gain weight and stay within your set point.

Nevertheless, should this behavior continue (eating too many calories), your body will interpret this as a signal to "re-set" to a new higher body weight range or "set point" over time. Unfortunately, many of us are very familiar with these bodily responses.

Eating too few calories...

Again, assuming you are currently within your set point, whenever you eat too few calories, your body has several mechanisms that start kicking in to slow things down and start conserving energy (calories).

Examples of things that will slow down or be reduced include:

- Your appetite increases above normal.
- Your metabolism (your whole "engine") starts slowing down and burning less.
- Your body's energy levels drop so you're less active and burn less calories. (It takes more effort to do just about everything.)
- You may feel lethargic.
- Your attitude may be significantly less positive (cranky).
- Your motivation to "do things" flat out disappears.

Again these and many other changes start immediately, and their purpose is to burn off less calories so that you can conserve energy (calories) and stay within your set point.

Your hormone profile will change, and just about everything you eat will immediately be stored as fat <u>even before</u> re-balancing other bodily functions.

To summarize, your body weight "set point" is a weight or fat percentage range that your body feels comfortable with. Your body will, through several mechanisms, resist going too far outside this range.

A quick note...

Your body and mind will "resist" increasing your body weight set point, but will aggressively FIGHT you if you try to lower it.

Why Does It Exist?

There are many reasons why we have a body weight set point. Two basic reasons are:

1. Survival!

Our bodies are designed for survival. One of the ways this is accomplished is by operating on the least amount of energy possible. This is accomplished by having many body systems or functions running on "auto pilot" within set ranges.

2. Works best!

Our body weight set point, along with hundreds if not thousands of other set points throughout our bodies, are designed so the whole system, our whole being, functions optimally.

It's All in My "Genes"...

When it comes to obesity, genetics are often the go-to scapegoat for many. We want to believe it's not our fault. Yes, there are genetic variants that can predispose us to higher or lower body weight set points, but their effects are small. Furthermore, epigenetic research indicates that certain "obesity genes" can be "turned off" through exercise alone. It's no surprise, then, that physical activity levels play a large role in determining our body weight set points.

What Influences Our Body Weight Set Point?

- Health
- What we regularly eat
- How much we regularly eat
- Our activity levels
- How much muscle we carry on our frame
- Our hormone profile
- Our cortisol levels (stress hormone)

- Inflammation
- Genetics
- Our constant internal conversations
- Our self-image

It should be mentioned here that many of the above work together or offset each other. For example, you can exercise every day until the "cows come home" and not lose a single pound because your appetite is programmed to increase in response. If you satisfy your appetite, you will negate most of your work. To simplify it all, it's the ongoing *relationship* between energy intake and energy output that influences your body weight set point.

Can It Be "Reset?"

YES, INDEED! This has been repeatedly shown, and we have all met someone that has taken the weight off and kept it off. However, there are only a few effective methods of resetting your body weight set point. The popular, ineffective ways are countless and often comical.

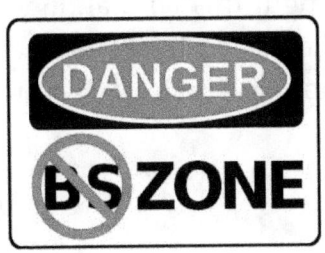

Effectively and permanently resetting your weight set point will take time. It will take very specific strategies and consistent effort. It requires knowledge, skill, and persistent attention during the process. You must be willing to begin stretching of your comfort zones. The reprogramming of your subconscious mind and adjusting of your self-image are key factors. All that said, it will be one of the most exhilarating experiences of your life.

Also, once you've mastered this skill, you can use the same process to "reset" any other area in your life.

How to Effectively Reset Your Body Weight Set Point

Again, FIRST and foremost... to effectively and permanently lower your weight set point will take time! There's just no way around that. How many YEARS has it taken to get where you are now? You cannot expect to lose it all in the next two months, at least not in a healthy and permanent way.

I know people fight this with all kinds of short term, misplaced confidence in the "latest" quack job or fad, but seriously, how has that worked out in the past?

So here's the bottom line:

"The faster you lose weight, the harder it will be and the lower your odds of success."

"The slower you lose weight, the easier it will be and the higher your odds of success."

Scientific research has proven time and again that the average person can lose approximately 10% of their body weight before they start running into aggressive resistance, before things start getting much more challenging and frustrating.

At that point you will have two choices:

#1 - Dig deep, find the resolve and continue.

#2 - Throttle back your efforts a bit and stay at this new weight for several months before moving to your next 10% target.

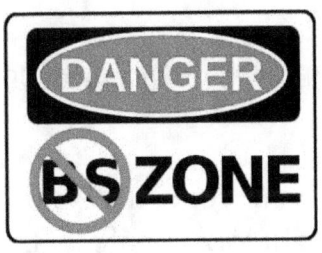

Real, repeatable, and confirmed scientific research has proven, without a doubt, that the most effective ways to "reset" your body weight set point is to drop approximately 10% of your body weight and hold it there for an extended period of time. Besides, if you can't maintain a 10% decrease in weight, what makes you think you will maintain more than this? So you MUST resist the urge to lose more. Again, has it ever worked before? You always end up putting it all back on. Being stubborn and losing more than 10% because "this time is different" will surely fail in the long run. Sorry, there's just no way around it.

How Much Time?

Although everybody is different, the most common successful time frame has been around six months. You don't have to wait six months, but remember that you always have the same two options available to you.

They remain the same…

- #1 - Dig deep, find the resolve and continue (start again).

- #2 - Throttle back your efforts a bit and stay at this new weight for several months before moving to your next 10% target.

Keep in mind that we are talking about "natural" and "healthy" weight loss. No drugs, no surgery, no balloons, etc. The "trick" is working with your body's natural tendencies to lose weight slowly rather than fighting against it. Take one step at a time, slowly, sustainably, and permanently.

Common Causes for Failure

What are the most common causes or reasons for failure to maintain your new, lower set point?

- Lack of focus
- Lack of motivation (not a big and clear enough "WHY", chapter one)
- Too far too fast, unable to maintain
- Unsustainable diet practices
- Unsustainable lifestyle
- Work (finances)
- Family members threatened and not supportive

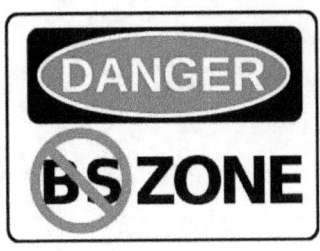

There are a hundred plus more "reasons" for failure but they are all B.S. They are all excuses. (Sorry, but it's true.)

Even if one didn't succumb to any of the seven reasons above, <u>if one fails to adjust their mental, habitual, and emotional set points,</u> failure is all but guaranteed. It's just a matter of time and succumbing to a trigger.

Also, a quick mention here... there are many other "set points" in our lives. Every one of them is affected by the others. You cannot drastically alter one without having a significant effect on the others. A 300-pound persons acts, thinks, responds, and LIVES differently than a 150-pound person. There is no doubt about that.

Pushing Your Limits

Are there ways to "push the limits" and fast forward resetting our body weight set point?

Yes, there are indeed!

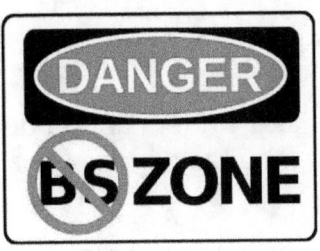

If you have a consistent and significant weight "issue," then the odds are that there are "issues" in one or more other areas in your life. These should be looked at, "fixed," and NOT used as excuses.

This is not the time for "patch-up jobs" and or "Band-Aid" solutions.

Excess weight is a result; it's a symptom of some other cause. If the causes are not properly addressed, then it will either be a lifelong struggle to maintain your new weight set point or something eventually will happen and cause failure. This is why I always advocate <u>working on several areas of your life at the same time.</u> In this way, you build very serious **MOMENTUM** in your whole life. The small successes that you build in each area are not "added," they are **COMPOUNDED** together to help move your life forward in the directions you seek.

"Your set points rule your world, and most can be adjusted to serve you."

Quick review...

What we know and understand about set points, especially our body weight set point:

- Our body has many of them.
- They are designed so that our body will run smoothly.
- They are also designed to save and conserve energy (efficiency).
- They vary between individuals.
- The non-life critical ones can be raised or lowered.
- When modified more than approximately 10% of our body weight, our body fights back.
- It is easier to raise them than it is to lower them.
- They are well within our personal control.
- Our total daily food intake has a strong effects on them.
- What we eat (nutrition dense vs. processed crap) affects it.
- Our consistent protein/carbs/fat ratio impacts them.
- Our lifestyle affects them.
- Our motivation levels matter a lot.
- Our inherited genes can have a small effects or lead to certain tendencies, but our upbringing has much more of an effect.

- Our hormone profile has a major impact on them.
- Our daily activity levels have a tremendous impact on them.
- The kind of activities we participate in affects them (high volume vs. high intensity).
- How much muscle we carry on our frames affects them.
- Our self-image affects them.
- Our stress and cortisol levels have a big effect on them.
- The people we hang around with have a large impact on them.
- Your attitude towards life has a huge impact on them.
- Our health affects them.
- Our type of employment affects them.
- The majority of the above factors are interrelated (changes in one causes others to compensate).

Ok, so now what do we do?

By the way, congratulations for staying with me up 'til now. It is said that less than 5% of the population purchases one book per year, and most rarely get half way through! So you are already way ahead of the masses, and you are starting to build some MOMENTUM. This is so critical!

Depending on where your self-image is at, part of your mind (sensing change and success) may already be starting to mount a defense. You will know this by the small little voices telling you that this is not for you, that you've tried everything in the past and that this too will fail, why even bother, that you're getting older and that it's normal to put on weight, that happiness is more important, etc., etc.

Don't be fooled for a second.

This is your time. Every past failure has laid a foundation for today. Every past failed attempt is being used as fuel that will propel you higher. THIS is the time. Today we do it properly and permanently. We start moving forward. Today we start building MOMENTUM.

(Following through with this will do absolute wonders for your self-confidence and your self-image. This will translate into many other areas of your life.)

Let's put it all together.

I'm assuming that:

- You are serious.
- You are doing this for yourself and no one else.
- That you ARE NOT just "trying" this; you will actually follow through.

- That you now understand why and how "weight set points" work.
- That you realise it took years to get here and it will take a bit of time to fix.
- That you are willing to take that time and do it properly and permanently.

A Simple But Very Effective Game Plan

#1 - Agree

To start off, you must agree that you will give your bodily systems, including your mind, all the time they need to adjust to your new 10% lighter body weight. If you're thinking, "We'll see how it goes…" then you are setting yourself up for failure. This measly 10% is NOT a huge amount, and that's one of the problems. People want to lose more, but losing more has never worked in the past, so what makes you think it will work this time? (**You will be able to lose more, but this will take special tricks, strategies, and more.**)

#2 - Contemplate

Next, sit down and think about what you are endeavoring to achieve. Really think about it. Don't sugar coat it. Realise that this will be challenging and uncomfortable, and that it won't happen overnight. Your hormones, emotions, and mind will be on a rollercoaster for a while. MORE IMPORTANTLY, understand that you are gradually moving closer and closer to the NEW YOU. The slimmer, healthier, more energetic, younger-looking, incredibly hot you.

#3 - Do the math

Next, do some quick math. Multiply your body weight by 10%, and that figure equals the target amount of weight to lose. (Body weight) x 10% = (Target).

#4 - Start exercising

Now that we have a target, the goal is to start increasing physical activity gradually **WITHOUT decreasing food intake!** The keyword here is gradually. If you're out of shape and go nuts right out of the gate, you may be in some serious pain for the next few days. This is enough to cause 30% of participants to quit. I say WITHOUT decreasing food intake because for the first week or two, just the increased activity will shock your system. Your body will instantly start moving toward your goal. Keep in mind that increased activity will speed up your metabolism and probably increase your appetite. I said not to decrease food intake, neither should you increase it.

#5 - Start reducing the pop

Immediately start reducing pop intake, including diet pop. I didn't say "all" pop. If you're drinking several cans a day, start by cutting one. Then next week, cut another one, and so on. Again, there are many biological, mental, and hormonal "set points" that will be affected by all the changes you are making. This includes reducing your pop intake! So going from three a day to none will start to freak your systems out by the third or fourth day.

#6 - Start replacing juices for water

However many weeks it takes is irrelevant, but <u>after</u> all the pop has been cut out, start to cut out all the other "glorified" juices. Replace these with water, and drink lots of it. This is a BIG move. You are slowly modifying your taste buds. If you're having trouble with the water change, just add lemon, lime, or even cucumbers. This seems to make it easier for many. These changes will do absolute wonders for your body even though your mind will start to fight you by the fifth day. Just be aware of it, "lean forward," and keep going.

#7 - Start cleaning up the serious garbage

Next, start decreasing your garbage intake. Candy, chocolate bars, chips, etc. If your intake of this crap is low, you may want to cut it out of your diet completely. However, if you're eating three chocolate bars a day, you may want to decrease gradually. Remember: this is all done gradually. Drastically changing your "food" intake will shock several of your systems, including your self-image, and may prove unsustainable. Notice that I don't give or set a time line. This should all be done very gradually and over time. At this point, you may be in week three or four already. Rushing the process will only guarantee failure. "I need to lose 20 pounds by next month for the wedding…" is NOT what we are going for!

Remember that you have been exercising throughout this time, preferably a mixture of basic cardio and resistance training. Nothing too hard and fancy.

#8 - A little less of the not so good crap

At this point, you are still maintaining your original amount of food intake calorie wise, more or less. I don't believe in counting calories nor measuring and weighing food portions. These practices are not sustainable. A rough guess is good enough. You are not a child. If you want to be stupid and accidently increase your food intake… hey, it's your life. Now #8 is to start slowly REPLACING "questionable" food with nutritiously dense foods. This time, I don't mean candy and stuff. I mean gradually start replacing pizza with salad, and lots of it. Another example, if you are eating out at fast food places three time a week, start cutting it back to two, then one, and eat at home more often.

By now, your diet should be pretty much all cleaned up. This may be week three or it could be week six! It all depends on where you were when you started. Again, the secret is to be slow, steady, and gradual. When done properly, this will translate into sustainable and permanent change. As we discussed in the section on habits and re-wiring the brain: we are gradually forming new neuro-associations, and these need time to "set" properly.

#9 - Gradually increase your greens

You should start to gradually increase your "greens" intake. When you have a salad, make sure it has plenty of broccoli, cauliflower, spinach, etc. Feel free to add a high quality, healthy oil rather than some crappy salad dressing. I know some people cringe at this, but again, are you serious or not? Eat lots of greens and as much of a variety as you can. You cannot eat too much. (Personally, I hate greens, so I don't skimp on the oil or vinegar I use. I do, however, make sure it is of the absolute best and healthiest quality.)

Remember that at this stage you still have not decreased your calorie intake! The increased activity, the switch from crap to healthy foods, and the resulting significant reduction in daily sugar intake will be enough to cause your weight to gradually drop.

#10 - Up the workout intensity

Next, start increasing the <u>intensity</u> of your workouts, but not the duration! So if you are training three or four times a week for 45 to 60 minutes, keep the time the same just increase the intensity (faster, heavier, harder, and more explosive). This is where we separate the men from the boys, the serious from the "I wish." You see, this is another "set point" or comfort zone. If you're jogging at a certain tempo, it's much easier to just maintain the tempo and run a little farther. That's what everyone does, and it works for a short time. However, you will then run into another set of problems. It is much more advisable to maintain the same amount of time and gradually increase the intensity. This will involve stretching your comfort zones.

If you've led a very sedentary lifestyle up to this point, your increased exercising (cardio and resistance training) will cause a pleasant change in your muscle tone. Your strength should have already increased by now, and this could mean a small increase in weight. Don't fret, this is the GOOD kind of weight. This is building up your calorie burning engine, which will gradually increase your metabolism. So DO NOT GET DISCOURAGED by a possible small weight gain. Besides, the mirror is your best friend, not the scale. I never stood on a beach and told my buddy, "Hey, check out that 134.5 pound girl!" In the grand scheme of things, how you look is what matters. You can have two 144 pound ladies stand side by side, and one looks hot and the other... not so much. So if you lost five pounds of fat and toned up five pounds of muscle on you glutes, etc., the transformation is awesome even if the scale says you haven't lost a single pound! The second best judge is how your clothes are not fitting. Third is how you're starting to feel.

When these processes are done honestly, the weight is already coming off. Nothing fancy here, but that's the secret. Most of the people who tend to be fit and healthy do not do anything superhuman. They just stick to the basics. It is NOT natural to weigh 300 pounds! Then again, it is not "natural" to sit all day and eat crap. Increase the activity (intensity), clean up your food intake, and improve your psychology. Nature will take care of the rest, and we'll cover that in the next chapter.

Keep in mind that there are over 30 "tricks" that can be used to help speed things up and increase your results. These are all covered in detail in a step by step guide coming out in a few weeks. See end of book for more information.

Here's one of the tricks: cut out all sugar and simple carbs after 7:00 pm. I won't explain why this is so powerful, but I will tell you it works and there are many others like it.

Chapter Five:
Your Subconscious Mind

Your Weight Loss Ticket Is Already Paid For

Remember:

"Life is won or lost in your mind FIRST."

"Change your mind, change your life."

Before We Start.

It would be well worth taking a few minutes to seriously ponder the following questions. These will lay a solid foundation on which we can then build a strong understanding of how our conscious mind works and how our subconscious mind literally control our entire life! Once we have a good grasp of this, only then can we move on and understand how we can control our subconscious mind, and thus our lives.

- Why do you procrastinate?

- What makes a person shy?

- Who "says" you can't do that thing you always wanted to?

- Always broke and living from paycheck to paycheck while many others making the same income do well and are steadily getting ahead?

- Are you always struggling with your weight and fitness, and why?

- Why are relationships a constant battle and often end up being "short term?"

- Why are some people generally positive while others are always negative?

- What makes life a "drag" or a "blast?"

- Why don't you think you can live the life of your dreams?

- Do you often catch yourself NOT following through on the best of your plans?

- Are you always struggling with mild food addictions or worse?

- Deep down, are you secretly afraid?

- Is your career going nowhere?

- Why are you NOT following your passions?

- Are you always eating "crap" when you know better?

- Are you still dragging old baggage that should have been dealt with a long, long time ago?

- Why don't you do what you know you should do?

The answers all lie in the deep recesses of your **SUB-CONSCIOUS** mind. It's time to adjust other thermostats in your life.

The Latest Research

A quick note here before we start getting into the thick of things. Much of the information about the brain, both the conscious and the subconscious minds, is outdated at best. If you're reading something that was written sometime before 1985, the odds are it is either completely wrong or at the very least, partially inaccurate. More has been discovered in the last 20 years than practically, well, ever. With the advent of new technology, especially the invention of MRI (magnetic resonance imaging), the ball has really started rolling on research regarding the brain. The MRI was quickly followed with even better technology, like PET scans (positron emission tomography), SPECT scans (single photon emission computed tomography), and so on. Today, we have technology that allows us to study and watch the brain react and work in **REAL TIME.** This has completely revolutionized what we understand about how our brains actually function. We have a much better knowledge of how the conscious and the subconscious mind work together but separately. We've learned far more about why many of us are held back from reaching our goals despite our best intentions. With all the new information available, it's become very clear what needs to be done in order to steer our lives in the direction we choose.

Our Brain

A few quick facts:

Our brain is by far the most complex piece of "machinery" on this earth. We are just beginning to "scratch the surface" of its capabilities. Having over 100,000 miles of blood vessels combined with over a hundred billion neurons. It can literally perform tens of millions of operations per second, every second of the day, and without getting tired! Every minute that we are alive, our brains oversee tens of millions of cells being dismantled, decommissioned, and done away with all while effortlessly creating equal amounts of completely new living tissue. Our brain manages and oversees literally millions of very specific and delicate "set points" (more on this later). Educating you on and detailing all of the intricate functions of the brain is not the purpose of this book, though. A quick Google search on the topic will open your eyes as to just how powerful the brain truly is. I will end with this fact: our brains represent a small 1-2% of our total body weight, yet it consumes about 20% of the oxygen we breathe, which is about the same for our blood flow. It uses up about 30% of all the nutrients from our blood, including 20% of all the water we drink. Remember, our brain is only 1-2% of our body weight!

One, Two, or Three Brains?

This is what we will be looking at. This is where, if understood and acted on, we can begin to make dramatic and positive changes in our lives.

Of course we don't have two or three brains, but we have two main "components." The difference between the two are night and day. They are the conscious mind and the subconscious mind, and they work together like a team despite the fact that their duties are vastly different. <u>Misunderstanding which mind performs what keeps people in their prisons.</u> Like the horse that is tied to a free standing plastic chair, we are often held captive to the smallest of mental strings. Regardless, like powerful steel cables, they hold us securely in a position of living far, far below our full potential.

Conducting the Music,
But Not Playing Anything

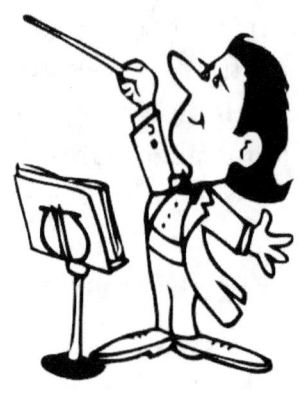

The conscious mind is like a conductor or director of a large orchestra. The conductor gives the orders and directs the musicians. He signals certain instruments to stop, start, slow down, speed up, move louder and more energetically, change the tempo, etc. He does all this with "cues" from his hand, arm, baton, and even visual "looks." The conscious mind is the part of our brain (frontal lobe or prefrontal cortex) that thinks, reasons, plans, decides, evaluates, concentrates, focusses, observes, learns, etc. It is the part that is reading this page. Our conscious mind is where we decide that we will lose some weight, start an investment portfolio, work on improving our relationships, work on overcoming shyness, etc. It's the boss... at least for a few minutes! Once it has given its orders, all the musicians (subconscious mind) handle the rest.

Caught in Our Own Illusions

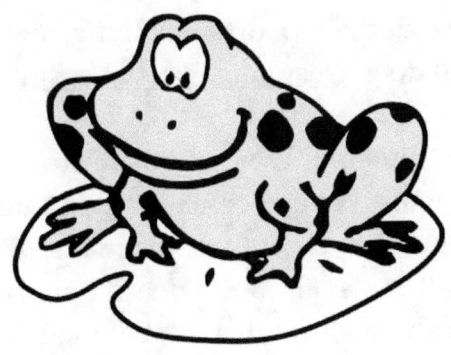

6 frogs sat on a lily pad.
1 decided to jump off.
How many are left?

- If I've decided to lose 20 pounds, why haven't I?

- If I've decided to start a savings or an investing plan, why haven't I?

- If I've decided to start a business, why haven't I?

- If I've decided to overcome my shyness, why am I still shy?

- Where did all my new year's plans go?

- Why am I pretty well where I was 5, 10, 15 years ago in my life?

See? That's the illusion. Just because the frog "decided" to jump off, doesn't mean that it actually did! Just because we decide to do something, doesn't mean that we will do it. <u>Despite our very best intentions.</u>

That's the illusion. We can plan, strategies, write down our goals. We can break it all up into nine easy steps, and put it in charts and diagrams. We can ponder the smallest details, but it doesn't matter. The part of the brain that does all this planning **is NOT** the part that actually follows through and makes sure things get done. And as long as "WE" (the conscious) think that "WE'RE" in charge, we will continue to live in our illusions and go absolutely NOWHERE.

<u>This is vital. This is absolutely critical. Without a clear understanding of which part of the mind handles what, we are doomed to a life that falls far short of our possibilities.</u> It doesn't matter how much you're serious this time. It doesn't matter that you really, really want it. It doesn't matter how many books you read or how many degrees you have. If you are depending on the wrong part of the brain to accomplish your goal, failure is inevitable.

There's just no room for flexibility here. Our brain does not work one way on Monday and a different way on Friday. It doesn't work one way for some and a different way for others.

I know I am repeating myself, but there's just no point in going any farther if you don't understand this.

Because we identify ourselves so strongly with the "conscious" part of our brain, we think that "it" is us! We think it is "us" that is reading this page. We think it is us that is setting and writing down the goal, that it is us that will do what it takes to reach it. BUT IT ISN'T.

Remember, we have both a conscious mind and a subconscious mind, and they are BOTH "us."

The question is not, "Can you?"

The question is, "Will you?"

There is no doubt that you can. The question is, "Will you?" This is why "knowledge" is not power. The "application" of knowledge is power. That is the difference between the doers and the readers.

We assume that it's our conscious mind calling the shots, but it's not. Not even close. Just like the conductor does not make any sounds (music) and only leads and guides, the conscious mind has very little to do with what gets accomplished.

Three Major Limitations
of the Conscious Mind

The conscious mind is critical for functioning properly. The conscious mind is where we "decide" what we want to do, where we want to go. This part of the mind gives us our creativity, and without that, we would go nowhere. Just like most brilliant and skilled orchestras cannot function properly without a conductor, or a corporation without its CEO, our "lives" cannot function without our conscious mind directing our subconscious mind.

> #1 - **Limited focus:** As important as our conscious mind is, it does have very serious limitations. For one, it cannot stay focused on any one task for very long. On average, we tend to lose focus every 20 seconds. Even though it's a very exciting and empowering feeling to be consciously directing our lives, it is but for a short time.

> #2 - **Limited memory:** The conscious mind is also limited in its ability to remember things. For example, if I randomly gave you 10 numbers, how many would you remember?

> #3 - **Cannot multitask:** Why is it illegal to drive and talk on a hand held device? Personally,

even if the phone is not hand held, I can't simultaneously drive normally and have a conversation (on a phone). Don't get me wrong. It's obviously doable, but my driving speeds go down, reaction times triple, and I fail to notice many things, etc. The conscious mind is not designed to multitask, at least not very effectively.

Just looking at these three limitations alone, how could the world achieve so much in the last 50 years? How can we, as individuals, live life to the fullest with these serious limitations? There must be more at play here. And there is. Much, much more, but before we look at our subconscious mind, let's go a little deeper within our conscious.

Conscious Mind

The good:

- It does the thinking, planning, and strategising.
- It is where visions and dreams are born.
- It makes decisions and sets our goals.
- It decides what is positive or negative.
- It decides what is true and what is a lie.
- It directs our focus in the past, present, and future.

- It critiques, questions, wonders, and reasons.
- It evaluates and makes new decisions.
- It gives us our willpower.
- It can "day dream" and create.
- It is the part of us that concentrates and "learns."
- It is the part of you that is reading this.
- It does not produce emotions.

The not so good:

- It has very short term focus and loses it as much as every 20 seconds.
- It has very limited memory and struggles to remember 10 digits.
- It cannot efficiently multitask.
- It is not involved in monitoring any of the systems that keeps us alive.

The Captain of the Ship

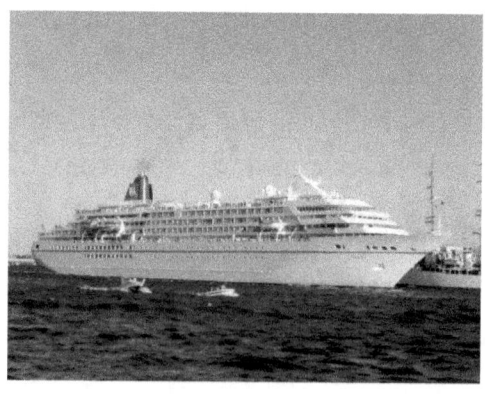

Again, the conscious mind operates like a captain directing a massive cruise ship. It is imperative that you understand the differences between the conscious and the subconscious minds, what they can and cannot do, and what they are responsible for. **Far too many are depending on the conscious mind to reach their weight loss goals,** their financial goals, and their social, family, business, fitness, everything goals. That's just NOT the responsibility of the conscious mind. Its responsibilities are more like the responsibilities of a ship's captain. The captain doesn't make the engines run harder so the ship can move faster. The captain doesn't control the cooling system to ensure the engine runs smoothly. On a typical cruise ship, there are over a thousand workers making sure EVERYTHING runs smoothly. The captain's job is to think things through, make decisions, and give orders.

The captain's job is to set goals. Just like the conscious mind's job is to think things through, make decisions, and set goals to direct your life. It is your subconscious mind's job to take orders <u>and follow through.</u> Just like employees complete what they are told without question, the subconscious does what it is told without question.

The captain does not sweep the floors, grease the engine, change the oil, gas up the ship, feed the crew, nor any of the other hundreds of tasks required for the ship to actually function. Just like you wouldn't expect the captain to perform these duties, neither should you expect your conscious mind to handle the hundreds or thousands of activities needed for you to reach your goals.

As the captain of the ship, your conscious mind has more important things to handle.

The Subconscious Mind and Endless Capabilities

In comparison, the subconscious mind is almost all powerful. It never sleeps, just like your heart never stops beating. If it did, you would immediately die. Your subconscious runs just about everything "behind the scenes," all without you being conscious of it. Think about that for a moment. Your subconscious mind keeps track of your body temperature, your breathing, your cellular water and electrolyte balance, your PH levels, and everything, trying to maintain a certain healthy range, or a "comfort zone."

Still, it's so much more than just that. Most of what we do in a typical day is habitual, **and it is the subconscious mind that "runs" all habits.** Have you ever eaten a meal while watching TV? Who was doing the "eating?" It most definitely was not your conscious brain. When the meal is over, can you remember "how" you ate, in what order, how fast, etc.? It was all habitual, and that's the job of the subconscious.

The conscious is heavily involved in LEARNING any new skills and knowledge. Consider learning how to drive a manual car. At first, it's hard. You keep stalling the engine when you engage the clutch. You forget to check your blind spot before turning. You're constantly going too fast or too slow. You can't maintain a conversation with your passenger, etc. Once you have learned the skill and rules, it all becomes a habit. The conscious is hardly involved anymore, other than deciding where to go. Your subconscious does the rest.

Now that your subconscious is involved, you get home after work, and you don't even remember how you got there! Who decided where to turn, which lane to be in, when to put the signals on?

When you catch a baseball, your subconscious mind does it all except "decide." Your conscious mind makes the decision, but the subconscious mind handles the action. Once you (conscious mind) decide to go for the ball, your subconscious decides the direction, how fast to take off, where the ball is going, at what speed, what is the descent rate, is there a strong wind, are there players or obstacles in the way, is the ground wet, muddy or slippery, when to extend your arm, etc., etc.

Think about it. There are hundreds of calculations being done in milliseconds. You just don't "take" a step! Which muscle fibers need to be activated, how many, what position to place the foot, etc. There are literally MILLIONS of calculations being done instantaneously without any effort.

That and so much more is all done, all the time, without any effort by our subconscious mind. All the conscious did was decide, "Yes, I will go catch the ball." All the conscious mind did was set the goal. The subconscious did all the rest.

And still, it's so much more. We have countless thought habits, feeling habits, reaction habits, and so on. When we meet a person for the first time, our subconscious does tens of thousands of calculations and within seconds you either feel "connected" or not.

Your conscious brain can barely remember an eight digit number, and if it does it will retain it for about 20 seconds. Your subconscious remembers EVERYTHING perfectly and permanently. Under hypnosis, patients clearly remember events that happened 50 years earlier, in complete detail, even going all the way back to when they were young children.

No wonder people set goals or plans and never reach them. The conscious mind's job is to "decide" or set the goal. It is the subconscious that reaches the goal. It's the conscious that decides to go catch the ball, but it is your subconscious that actually does all the rest including catching the ball.

You may decide to "lose 20 pounds and get in shape," but it is your subconscious that does ALL THE REST. Deciding does not make it so. Deciding to jump off the lily pad does not mean you jumped. It doesn't even mean that you will ever jump.

If we don't understand how to engage our subconscious mind, we are destined to stay EXACTLY where we are in life. Why? Because that's the very job of our subconscious mind, the most powerful piece of technology in our universe bar none. Its job is to keep us in our comfort zones, in our habits. It does all this **because that's what we have repeatedly told it.**

Remember, the conscious mind determines what's right and what's wrong. What we want and what we don't want. What is positive and what is negative. What is true and what is not. The conscious mind calculates, evaluates, plans, concludes, identifies, analyses, etc. The conscious mind gives the orders just like the gardener decides which seeds to plant, but the earth or the garden is what makes everything grow.

The subconscious mind does not decide, it doesn't know the truth, can't draw conclusions, etc. It depends on the conscious mind to perform these tasks and to be accurate. It only does what it is told based on EVEYTHING, all inputs including the repetitiveness and emotions that go along with these orders. Your conscious mind can look to the past, the present and the future. <u>Your subconscious only "knows" the present.</u>

Your conscious mind decides what to focus on. Your subconscious mind makes it happen.

What Grows the Crop?

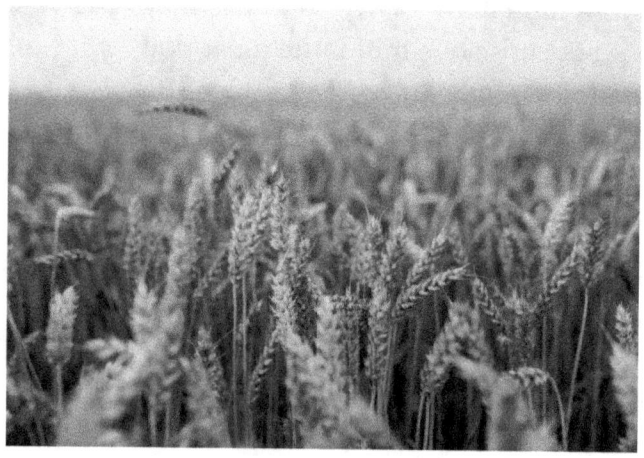

What grows the harvest? The farmer receives a lot of the credit, and if it wasn't for him, there definitely would be no crop. However, if you watch the whole process, and you see that other then planning, making decisions, and possibly being involved in the actual planting, the farmer has little to do with the actual "growing" or production of the crop. Nature does it all. How far would the farmer get without oxygen to feed or oxyginate the plants? Hundreds and thousands of biological processes require oxygen to produce complete growth. There would be no growth without oxygen. How many biological proccesses require sunlight to work efficiently or work at all? Could there be ANY growth without the sun? How about water? We've all had plants that we've forgotten to water before leaving the house for the weekend. What happens? Thousands of biological processes require water, and without it, NOTHING would happen. Lastly, what about the earth itself? All the various minerals and compunds plants need to grow? Even hydroponics requires "nutrients" in the water for the plants to grow.

This all sounds elementary, and you'd have to be half asleep not to know and understand these things. However, our conscious and subconscious minds work the same way. Our conscious mind's job is to pounder, think, analyse, decide, plan, and set "goals" for our lives. Where we want to go, be, do, or have. The conscious mind is the farmer. Our subconscious mind is the air, sun, water, earth, and all the labourers.

So WHY do we expect our conscious mind to reach our goals?

Subconscious Mind

The good:

- It monitors and oversees the tens of millions of body processes.
- It monitors and controls the body's "set points" or "ranges."
- It believes what it is repeatedly told as fact and truth.
- It is where our emotions are found.
- This is where all our physical and mental habits are stored.
- This the part of our brain that follows through on the thousands of actions needed to reach your goals (including weight loss).
- It never stops working.

The not so good:

- It doesn't think, question, conclude, analyse, decide, plan, direct focus, startegise, set goals, choose, give orders, etc.
- It can be hard to access and influence directly.
- It can be slow to change or influence.

- It can "seemingly" act contrary to our wishes.
- It won't forget.
- It never stops working.

Operates like: a corporations's thousands of employees following instructions and making things happen. The earth in the garden making and growing the plants. A massive orchestra following the conductors every command. The crew on a cruise ship making it run smoothly just how the captain has comanded.

By now you understand that the "captain" actually has little to do with the cruise ship reaching it's destination, or that in the grand scheme of things, the farmer also has very little to do with the crop actually GROWING.

It should also be starting to become obvious just how little our conscious minds are involved in actually following through and doing what needs to be done to reach our goals.

Without a good and thorough understanding of the different responabilities of the conscious and subconscious minds, reaching any worthwile goal can prove to be a complete waste of time.

So one last time, the conscious mind is like the CEO of a big corporation. He thinks, focuses, learns, analyses, ponders, critiques, questions, strategises, visualizes, etc. Finally, he makes decisions!

The subconscious mind is like the thousands of employees that "make it happen!" It really is that simple.

If we task our conscious minds with what it is NOT designed to do, nor can even begin to do, we will forever struggle and fail to reach our goals. The life that we envisioned will never come to pass just as the captain couldn't reach the planned destination without the crew.

You can decide to lose that 20 pounds, to start that bussiness, to overcome your shyness, to advance your career, to beat the negative self talk... but unless you involve your subconscious mind, you are wasting your time. "It" is the water, earth, sun, and oxygen that makes your goals grow and come to life. I hope this has become clear to you.

Now a few more tid bits, and then let's have a look at an example of what the subconscious mind can do.

Tid Bits

	Conscious	Subconscious
Brain mass	17%	83%
"Life" control	2%-10%	90% to 98%
Memory	short term (30 sec)	permanent
Impulse speed	130 mph	100,000 mph+
Proc. power	2,000 bits/sec	300 billion bit/sec
Time	past, present future	present

Now, let's look at a quick example of how the conscious mind and the subconscious mind are involved in reaching one simple goal.

To Catch a Baseball...

The conscious mind:

- The goal: I want to win the game.
- The sub-goal: I want to catch that ball.
- The decision: "go catch the ball."
- The focus: "go catch the ball."...

That's it! The conscious mind's job is pretty well done. It will observe, and it may make minor decisions here and there, but its only job is to think, plan, and decide.

(I have greatly simplified this whole example. If I didn't, it would take a whole encyclopedia just to list some of what the subconscious mind does to catch the ball.)

The subconscious mind:

The order: Go catch the ball. (Remember, the subconscious mind does not do the analysing, planning, and deciding. It only takes orders. It doesn't even question those orders. It takes them as truth. It's only job is to do what it has been told to do.)

Order received!

(It is the subconscious mind talking below.)

What is a ball? I will quickly scan my lifetime database. It comes up with the "correct" definition. (Remember there are many different kinds of balls, and they all react and travel at different speeds. You may think this is foolish, but how is the clump of "jelly" in your head even supposed to know what a ball is?)

Where is the ball? Actually, where am I? Oh yes, I'm at a baseball game. I just heard the "crack" of a bat hitting a ball. Based on the difference between the sound arriving at my two ears and the difference between the two, I can tell the sound is coming from this general area. Based on all the "bat cracks" I've heard through the years, I'd say this was a good one so the ball should be traveling at approximately "this" speed. Based on the time of the crack (figuring out the "time" is a whole other complicated process), the ball should be approximately here. I can now see it. I was wrong, it seems to be traveling roughly at "this" speed. It should be going faster? Why? Based on my database, the other times this has happened there was a head wind involved! There must be a wind. Yes, today it is windy, and the wind is coming from the east. I can see that the ball is coming down at "this" rate of descent. With the head wind, it will be slowing its forward speed even faster... at "this" rate, and it should be increasing its descent speed by "this" amount. Taking everything else into account, and their **INTER-RELATIONSHIPS** (there are dozens of other variables that need to be taken into account), I figure the ball will fall somewhere around there.

Now, how much time do I have to get from here to there and catch the ball before it lands on the ground? Based on my recent physical and biological performances, I figure I can get there in time. I think I will need a blast of specific hormones (a book can be written here alone on hormones) to help ensure my performance. I think I will also immediately re-route some of the blood circulation, glucose, and chemical balance in certain cells (another book).

Now for the first step! How much explosive pressure should I employ? Which leg should I start with? How far forward should I lean to counter act the take-off force so I don't fall backward? Okay, think I got it. Now which muscles should I use? Let's start with the calf. Do I even need the calf? Based on my database, it seems when I employ the calf muscles I get more leverage and thrust from my toes and feet. But wait, I've fallen before! Is the ground pavement? Is it gravel? Loose or packed? Is it wet grass? What type of shoe am I wearing?

Wow! Get the point? We haven't even taken the first step yet. The subconscious mind is still figuring out how much thrust to use based on the conditions of the ground! Next is how to coordinate the 26 bones, 33 joints, 107 ligaments, 19 muscles and tendons in one foot! Even if we just started with only one of the 19 muscles, how many fibers should we "fire?" Which ones should we "fire?" How will this combination affect the next joint? (Remember there are 33 joints just in one foot!)

To properly calculate all the variables is astronomical. Remember, it's **NOT** 2+2... 33 times (33 joints) = 68. The calculations are **exponential**. In other words it's 2x2... 33 times, and it's NOT 68, but instead it's 8,589,934,592! Now multiply that by 107 ligaments! I wasn't kidding when I said it would take a complete set of encyclopedia's to list all the actions needed to be performed and the millions of lightning fast calculations needed just to go catch a baseball. **Our subconscious mind does it all accurately and effortlessly all day long.** Contrast that to our conscious mind that loses focus every 20 seconds or so, that can't remember ten or so numbers, and cannot multitask more than two or three basic simple actions (and even messes those up). The subconscious does 99% of the work!

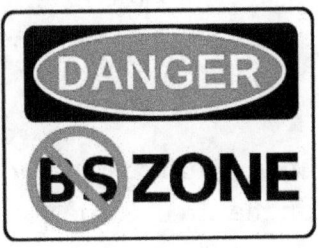

Depending on our conscious mind to reach ANY of our goals is completely futile! Yet, that's what most people try every year, all the time. They think that because they have decided to lose some weight that they will. Not a chance. (I'm talking PERMANENT weight loss.) Without effectively influencing your subconscious mind, reaching any of your goals will be a losing battle. It isn't Microsoft's CEO (conscious mind) that's making the billions. It's the tens of thousands of employees (subconscious mind). It isn't the cruise ship captain (conscious mind) that is making the ship run smoothly, it's the thousand workers (subconscious mind). It isn't "you" (conscious mind) that will successfully and permanently lose the weight, it's your SUBCONSCIOUS! (Again, I'm talking permanent weight loss.)

Your RAS (Reticular Activating System)

RAS, your reticular activating system, is the scientific term used for a network of nerve pathways at the base of your brain. It acts as a filter for all your sensory inputs coming in from the external world. There are tens of thousands of bits of information coming in every second.

Hearing: How many different sounds can be heard when standing on the street corner?

Touch (skin): How many "inputs" are coming in just from all the small hairs on your arm if you focused on that area?

Taste: How many taste buds are on the tongue alone?

Smell: How many odor receptors are in your nose, and how many different odors are there at any one time?

Eyesight: You can't even begin to count all the objects our eyes pick up in 60 seconds.

These inputs are all coming in at the same time and continuously.

If it wasn't for the RAS, our conscious mind would overload instantly. Making decisions would be impossible.

The purpose of the RAS is simple:

It filters out the stimulus **we have deemed unimportant.** It manages our "sense perception." It is a kind of "gatekeeper." It acts as a "goal seeking" mechanism. The RAS determines what information gets through to you, what you notice, what grabs your attention. **It also prevents you from noticing EVERYTHING else.**

Simply put, what you value gets through, what you devalue gets filtered out.

Three examples of how the RAS works:

#1 - It is a bright, warm, sunny day. You're sitting at a popular playground. Your kids are playing along with dozens of other children. There is never-ending laughter, yelling, screaming, etc. Add to that parents calling out to their kids, dogs barking, continuous traffic on the streets, etc. You are sitting nearby reading a book. Anybody else would not be able to make out your daughter's voice but should something happen, even while you are engrossed in your book, you would instantly hear her yell and respond.

#2 - You're sound asleep. The TV is playing in the next room. Traffic is honking and constantly rumbling by. Dogs are barking. None of that bothers you as you sleep soundly. All of a sudden your infant makes the slightest unusual sound, and you are up instantly.

#3 - You just purchased a blue truck. On your way to work you can't help but notice how many other blue trucks are on the road.

This is your RAS filtering out all the unimportant and letting through what we value.

How can we best use our RAS to help us reach our goals?

We can start by having **clearly defined** goals. (Remember the first chapter, the second dynamo, "Clarity"). Only by spending quality time determining what is truly important to us, what we are committed to achieving and why, will our RAS perceive it as VALUABLE and IMPORTANT. From this point, all sensory inputs related to your goal or whatever you are focused on will be brought to your attention .You will "notice" it. Your RAS will also deem it valuable and let it go through its filters. The critical condition here is "clarity." Your goals must be crystal clear.

A quick personal example:

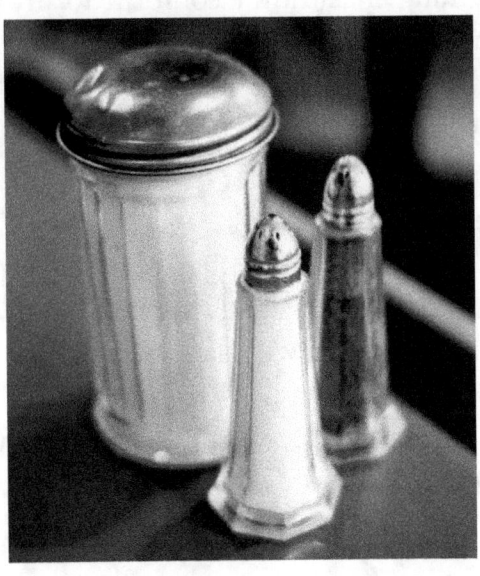

I was recently in Niagara Falls enjoying lunch with my wife in a beautiful restaurant. About to enjoy our coffee, she asked if I would pass the sugar. I started to oblige, but I couldn't find it. There was an odd silence as she looked at me in bewilderment as I just "stared" at the sugar. The thing was, I couldn't see any sugar. I sat there staring right at the sugar, but I could not see it. She wondered if I was joking around. You see, that morning we had breakfast at IHOP, and the sugar was in a glass bottle. So when she asked me for sugar, my brain started scanning for a glass bottle of sugar. Just 15 inches in front of my face was a container filled with sugar packets, yet I could not see any sugar whatsoever on the table! Then I noticed how she was looking at me, like "duh," and looked again. There it was as plain as day. My RAS was filtering out everything that didn't conform to my "picture" (goal) of what I was looking for.

Setting Goals

We understand that despite what many think, it is NOT the conscious mind that reaches our goals in life, but it is the subconscious mind. Going back to the very beginning where we talked about "decisions" (in Chapter One, "Weight Loss Prison section"), we understand that the conscious mind, the part that thinks, plans, strategizes, and decides, is the part that makes decisions and sets the goals. The conscious mind decides to "catch the ball" (set the goal), and the sub-conscious does the hundreds or thousands of minor actions that culminate in reaching the goal of catching the ball.

This is not a goal setting book, so we will just briefly touch on the subject. Goal setting in itself is a great exercise, but without involving the subconscious, it ends up being a waste of time. We will come back to this in a few pages.

Successful goal setting should always start with a good mental stretching exercise. By that, I mean it should start with a "dream" list. A dream list is where you write down EVERYTHING you even "think" you may want to be, do, or have. This list should be written fairly fast with absolutely NO questioning or judgements of any kind. If you "think" you "might" then write it down.

Next, break them up into three categories:

> #1 - Short range goals (one year or less)
> #2 - Medium range goals (one to five years)
> #3 - Long range goals (five years or more)

Choose the four that are the most important to you. Research has shown that we can only effectively work on a small handful of goals at any one time. These goals should be "balanced," meaning they should not all be financial or material. A happy and successful life must be balanced, so there should be material, career, family or relationships goals, etc.

Now that you've chosen your four most important goals, the following step is to "list the major obstacles and challenges to reaching these goals." Do not skip this or any of the next steps. They are all necessary and dramatically increase the odds of you reaching your goals. Listing the major obstacles will open your eyes to things you may not have taken into consideration or you will need to know about later.

Now, "list all the skills or knowledge required to reach these goals." Again, are you serious about reaching these goals? Then follow through and complete all the steps.

Next, "list a minimum of ten benefits of reaching these goals." Let's face it. Some of your goals will prove to be quite challenging, and if you don't have a solid understanding as to WHY you are doing all this work, you run a good chance of failing.

The last step is fun. The conscious brain is heavily involved as you, "list the plan of action to reach these goals." Go nuts here and strategize as best you can. A lot of these strategies will have to be modified along the way, but that doesn't matter right now.

Properly done, you can expect to spend several hours on setting your goals. It involves a lot of thought. Many people will go at great lengths to avoid having to think at all, so is it any wonder that many never reach their full potential? Having followed through here has placed you in the top 5% of the population. Remember, a goal that is NOT written down and set properly is just a dream that's completely devoid of any power. It will most likely not even launch.

Please contact me if you would like the "Seven Step Goal Setting Worksheets."

Reaching Goals

This is where you enter the "big leagues." Everything you want in life and all achievements are found here. Unfortunately, this is also where many completely blow it as they constantly fight against themselves.

To explain, the conscious mind has set the goal, but the subconscious mind is not in agreement. In a fit of determinations, will power, and temporary clarity, the conscious mind has made a decision and has set a specific goal. "I want to lose 20 pounds." Most likely, this is being done on a Monday morning. By coffee time we're already blowing it. "Hmm, boy I'd love to have that donut along with my coffee, but <u>I'm 30 pounds overweight</u>..." By lunch time, they have already contradicted themselves many times. It continues when they decide what to have for lunch. "Hmm, I'd love some of that pizza, but <u>I'm fat.</u> I said I wanted to lose some weight..." Between lunch and dinner, many other opportunities will arise as they mentally (or verbally) tell themselves (or their friend) that <u>they are fat</u>... This goes on hour after hour, day after day, week after week for years.

So what is happening? Hopefully by now you understand that it is your subconscious mind that reaches your goals (catches the ball). It is NOT your conscious mind. The subconscious mind only deals with the present tense, the NOW. When you set a goal by saying, "I want to lose 20 pounds," it doesn't "compute." Your subconscious mind says, "Okay, so what?" To make matters so much worse, by the end of the day you have told it, "I AM fat" a hundred times! In the PRESENT and with EMOTIONS!

At the end of the day, which command do you think your subconscious mind will believe? The one time statement "I want to lose 20 pounds," which not being in the "now" doesn't even register? Or the hundreds of times you told yourself, "I'm fat" in the present tense and with emotions? Of course it will fully accept the latter as the command and the truth in which to operate. After all, you've been telling it like you mean it (emotions) many times over throughout the day, every day, for years now. Your subconscious mind, which does not question but only accepts and acts on what it is told, will do everything in its CON-SIDERABLE power to make your command come true. The command you repeatedly told it: "I am fat."

All of the thousands of body functions and processes are monitored and controlled by your subconscious mind. There are literally tens of thousands of "set points," or "ranges," or "comfort zones" that the sub-conscious mind is responsible for maintaining. Your body weight is just one of them.

At its disposal are hundreds of things it can do so that your body stays within its body weight range. All of these are done every day and without your conscious knowledge.

Your subconscious mind, in all of its power, <u>is follow-ing your commands perfectly all the time.</u> It's your subconscious mind that picks your vehicle, picks your clothes, picks your friends, etc. It controls every-thing. You, however, control IT. Knowingly or un-knowingly, it doesn't matter. You have the power at all times. Most, by default have given that power over to everything and everyone else. Don't you agree that it's time to take back control?

Next, we will look at a few very effective and basic ways to successfully influence and guide our subcon-scious mind.

Are you ready?

Neuroplasticity

(Purposely kept brief, simple, and short.)

Neuroplasticity is a general term used to describe the brain's ability to reorganise and transform itself by growing countless new neural connections and pathways every day until we die. The idiom, "You can't teach an old dog new tricks," was done away with about 20-plus years ago with the advent of new technology that allows scientists to study the brain more accurately and on a "live" or "real time" basis. For example, we have come to learn that the brain continuously builds, strengthens, and modifies countless neural pathways every day (neurogenesis). We also know that "neurons that fire together, wire together," and that this goes a long way in explaining how habits become habits, how they can become addictive and very hard to resist (Chapter 3). Luckily, we have also learned that it's just as simple to develop "good" habits as it is to develop "bad" habits. **Our daily habits ARE THE STRONGEST DETERMINING FACTOR of our ultimate destinies in life,** so perhaps we should spend a bit more time in learning how to successfully modify them to our advantage. This all starts with the brain.

Neuro Conditioning

(Purposely kept brief, simple, and short.)

Neuro conditioning (neural reconditioning) is a process by which we effect real, physical changes in our brains that serve to help us move closer and closer to our goals.

Before we get into the "good stuff," let me tell you about one experiment NASA did several years ago that illustrates the potential of what our brains are capable of achieving. This knowledge was proven with the advent of new technologies like the MRIs, PET scans, SPECT scans, MEG scans, etc.

NASA's Research:

In the 80s, NASA wanted to research how astronauts would handle zero gravity, including their balance and being "upside down" for extended periods of time in space. In this research, several astronauts volunteered to wear specially designed goggles with convex lens that made it appear as if their world was upside down. (I get a headache just thinking about it!)

They were required to wear their goggles 24/7 for 30 consecutive days.

Something totally unexpected happened along the way.

After between 26 and 30 days, every astronaut was seeing their world right side up again! We now know and understand that their brains had created enough new neural pathways to be able to turn the upside-down images that came through their eyes right side up. Their brains apparently did this so they could function more effectively!

In repeated trials, the researchers also discovered that if the astronauts took their goggles off at any time BEFORE the 30 days was finished, they had to start over completely.

The conclusion?

The brain can be significantly "re-wired." To effect changes, 26 to 30 days must pass uninterrupted.

Consistency is key.

Okay. It's our conscious mind that thinks, plans, and sets the goal, and that it's the subconscious mind that does everything else and makes everything actually happen. We also know that we can't just change "our minds" overnight and undo years of programing. Our subconscious mind's duties are so critically important and necessary for our very survival that it is not easily accessible. However, there are a number of effective ways of accessing and reprograming it so that it best serves our new direction.

Don't be fooled. There are no free lunches. Although many have and are continuously enjoying great success with these and other similar strategies, persistence, time, and effort will be needed to effect change. Years and often decades of continuous programing can seldom be changed overnight, but the process still works and works very well.

Why the strategies are so simple...

The strategies are very simple because that is how the brain works. You acquired your <u>current</u> beliefs, comfort zones, and self-image the same way. You were "brain washed" to believe your current limiting beliefs by constant negative self-talk (in adulthood), and you may have heard and seen it as a child. Obviously it's a bit more complicated than that. Complete brain washing involves all the senses, repetition, and emotions.

To delete, change or modify your past programing, <u>we need only use the exact same process.</u> Now that you understand how the conscious and subconscious minds work, we can begin to "download" better and more empowering belief systems, beliefs that will move you towards your goals instead of away from them. It's time to put an end to all the self-sabotaging.

Again, the process is very simple. We will use several of the exact same methods that you repeatedly used in the past to gain your current belief systems.

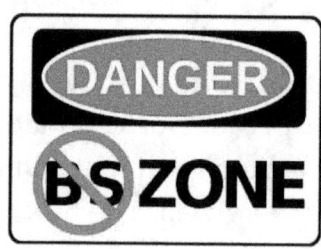

The problem, and the danger, is not that it's too hard, too expensive, too complicated, etc. The only problem is that it's too SIMPLE, and that you may not actually follow through. If you don't, you might as well "accept" your lot in life because if you are not willing to change, neither will your life.

The Strategy

Affirmations

If you have a significant weight challenge (your fat), the odds are extremely high that you have been telling yourself "this" over and over for many years in many different ways and situations. We will simply take control of it and just reverse it. **Start by making a**

<u>**simple, short, present tense, and positive affirmation.**</u> It should also be in the realm of possibilities for you. If you have been an extreme introvert and tentative person all your life, affirming that you are all powerful and unstoppable will be laughed at by your subconscious.

Examples:

- I am slim, trim, and fit. (Unless you have weighed 350 pounds for the last several years. Doable, but it may not be believable enough at first.)
- I am gradually losing weight every day.
- I am looking better and better every day.
- I exercise every day.
- I am eating better and better all the time.
- I weigh ___ pounds.

Come up with something that you can identify with and that "means" something to you. Keep them short, positive, present tense, and believable. Come up with several of them.

The next step is to INTERNALIZE them. This takes persistent effort and time. The good news is that it's very simple. The bad news is that it's very simple! Now that you have your affirmations, they must be said repeatedly, preferably out loud, preferably with emotions, preferably with physical activity, and at a bare minimum, for 30 days.

No way! Can it be that simple?

Simple YES, easy NO.

This is how you acquired your current limiting beliefs (including "I'm fat"), and this is how you will replace them. There are just no free lunches.

There are several things you can do that will help speed things up and generate quicker results. We will briefly go through them. They all revolve around using all your senses.

Saying: Say your affirmations out loud as often as you can. When you are sitting and consciously thinking about them, say them. Say them while you are doing something else, like jogging or other repetitive tasks. This will make your subconscious more accessible and deliver a bigger impact.

Visualizations (pictures): All the senses impact the subconscious mind, so if you're looking for a fitter, thinner, and healthier you, you should set up a binder with many pictures of body types that motivate you to reach your goal. You should look at them often and daily. Ideally, you will reach the point where you close your eyes and you can see the pictures. The absolute best time to do this is first thing in the morning and last thing at night. Make it more powerful by saying your affirmations while doing all this.

Writing: Writing out your affirmations while you are saying them will add considerable impact. The very act of writing them involves the subconscious to a much larger degree. (Extreme simplification!)

Reading: Have copies all over the house. Read them slowly, preferably while looking at pictures that exemplify your goal. Read with emotion. Read them often.

Listening: Make a recording of yourself reading or saying these affirmations out loud with emotion. Listen to them attentively and also in the background without paying attention. These are two distinct modalities. One involves the conscious mind, and the other involves your subconscious.

Meditation: To keep things simple, let's treat meditation just like day dreaming. Instead of day dreaming about useless things that will probably never happen, day dream (meditate) on the new you. Replace all counter-productive worrying with intentional day dreaming. Keep in mind that the more "real" you can make your day dreaming, the larger the impact on your subconscious mind.

Summary

Permanent weight loss is definitely doable. It is being done every day, and it can be done by you. Actually, it's quite simple. It's not easy, but it is simple. If we resist looking for short cuts and are willing to do what has to be done, then success is simply a matter of time.

*** WARNING ***

BE CAREFUL

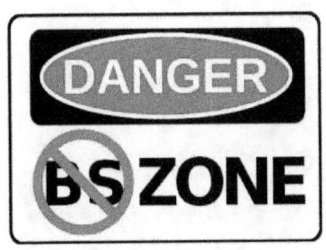

If you just whizzed through the last two sentences, you have either thoroughly studied and know the material, or you have greatly underappreciate just how "loaded" those statements actually are. The whole process is very simple, but that's the problem. It's often easy to dismiss parts of the formula. For example, take the first step, "I want to lose weight, and I will start Monday." That is a decision, but it completely misses what is explained in the first chapter.

You NEED to "get" and truly understand that the process ONLY works when done properly. You also need to "get it straight" that you've already tried just about everything, most likely several times, and one last time, HOW'D THAT WORK OUT FOR YA? You're probably worse off than at any other time. Do yourself a favor. No games, no short cuts, and no "half-ass" measures. After all, it's your LIFE that we're talking about. Start at the beginning of the book and follow each step in detail. When you start the "reprograming" of your limiting beliefs, remain patient. It takes a lot of effective repetition and time, at least 30 consecutive days. But it works every time.

I wish you wisdom.

Your coach,

Ray Blais

*** Bonus ***

There's so much more I'd like to give you. Unfortunately I need to keep this book fairly short or many would never purchase and benefit from it, much less read it.

Let me leave you with another one of those 30-plus nice simple tricks used by many successful people. It works extremely well and in so many different areas of life. Right now, I will stick with the weight loss theme and continue a bit more with our subconscious mind.

By now, I'm sure you have a good understanding that it's our subconscious minds that rule our lives! It is by effectively guiding our subconscious in the direction we wish to go that we can truly design the life we want. Unfortunately, it sometimes remains persistently unresponsive. Often, we can "feel" and "know" that it is fighting against us.

The trick is to get it to "play" with us and not try to force it. When you ask yourself a question, your mind will immediately start answering. <u>It cannot do otherwise</u>. Ask yourself why you are fat, and it will quickly tell you why. Ask yourself why you are sad, and again it will tell you why. Try it. It's surreal. You can almost hear your brain answer you. Unfortunately, this also happens when you are using affirmations that may be stretching the truth a bit too much. If you weigh 300 pounds and haven't exercised in years, try saying, "I'm a young, healthy, fit man!" You can almost hear your brain laugh! Therefore, your affirmation will be useless and quite possibly counterproductive.

So how do we get our subconscious to "play ball" with us? We start by asking strategic questions. Continuing with the 300 pounds out of shape person that's trying to put all this together, what would happen if instead of using an inappropriate affirmation, you asked something like, "Why am I feeling better today?" Listen to what your mind answers. It will go something like this, "Well, it's because you only had one pop instead of the usual four per day. It's because you now go for a walk every morning. It's because you now eat a salad every day, etc." **Your mind is now supporting you**. It's agreeing with you. It's backing you up instead of laughing and fighting with you. Try it.

Do this whenever you catch yourself performing below your potential. Next time you're cranky, don't say, "Why am I so miserable?" Your mind will quickly find ten reasons why, and you'll only feel worse. Instead, ask, "Why am I feeling a bit more relaxed today?" Listen! It will say things like, "Well, your favourite song is playing," or, "Earlier today that person was nice to you," or, "Look outside. It's so nice and sunny!" Your mind cannot resist. It will answer your questions.

Now all you have to do is **start asking the right questions** more often.

This alone can be transformational.

Do the NIKE thing... "Just do it!"

Conclusion

Finally, for those that wish to maximise their chances of success, here are additional ways we can continue to help you:

- **FREE Summary map and flow-chart** listing all the critically important points and steps covered in this book to be followed in the correct order for the quickest and best results.

- **FREE Special newsletter** designed strictly to inform, educate, and guide. No sales crap, no fluff, and no B.S. The "Fit" newsletter...

  LOOK GOOD – FEEL GREAT – STAY HAPPY

  o **30++ Tricks and Strategies** coming soon.

  o **Website:** http://familykickboxing.net

  o **Website:** https://www.facebook.com/FamKick/

  o **Email:** getfit@familykickboxing.net

I look forward to hearing from you.
Together, we can do this.
Ray

www.ingramcontent.com/pod-product-compliance
Lightning Source LLC
Chambersburg PA
CBHW071357310526
45789CB00020B/443